Clinical Management of Pulmonary Arterial Hypertension

First Edition

Editors

James R. Klinger, MD
Division of Pulmonary
Sleep and Critical Care Medicine
Rhode Island Hospital
Professor of Medicine
Alpert Medical School of Brown University

Alan Fein, MD, FACP, FCCP, FCCM
Clinical Professor of Medicine
Hofstra Northsore-LIJ School of Medicine
Chief, Pulmonary, Critical Care and Sleep Medicine
Prohealthcare Associates

Arunabh Talwar, MD, FCCP
Professor of Medicine
Hofstra North Shore-LIJ School of Medicine
Director, Advanced Lung Disease Center
North Shore-LIJ Health System

D1153906

COMMUNICATIONS, INC.

Professional Communications, Inc.

A Medical Publishing & Communications Company

400 Center Bay Drive
West Islip, NY 11795
(t) 631/661-2852
(f) 631/661-2167

1223 W. Main St, #1427
Durant, OK 74702-1427
(t) 580/745-9838
(f) 580/745-9837

For orders only, please call
1-800-337-9838
or visit our website at
www.pcibooks.com

ISBN: 978-1-932610-97-0

Printed in the United States of America

DISCLAIMER
The opinions expressed in this publication reflect those of the authors. However, the authors make no warranty regarding the contents of the publication. The protocols described herein are general and may not apply to a specific patient. Any product mentioned in this publication should be taken in accordance with the prescribing information provided by the manufacturer.

This text is printed on recycled paper.

TABLE OF CONTENTS

Editorial Assistance

Sara L. Merwin, MPH
Research Associate
Department of Orthopaedic Surgery
Long Island Jewish Medical Center
Assistant Professor, Medicine and Orthopaedic Surgery
Hofstra North Shore-LIJ School of Medicine

Contributing Authors

Steven Y Chang, MD, PhD
Associate Clinical Professor of Medicine
Pulmonary & Critical Care Medicine
David Geffen School of Medicine at UCLA

Daniel Green, MD
Assistant Professor of Radiology
New York-Presbyterian Hospital
Weill Cornell Medical College

Hussam Inany, MD
Third Year, Chief Resident
Department of Pediatrics
New York Methodist Hospital

Jason M. Lazar, MD, MPH, FACC, FACP
Professor of Medicine
Director, Non-Invasive Cardiology
Director, Cardiovascular Medicine Fellowship Training Program
SUNY Downstate Medical Center

Pramod Narula, MD
Chairman, Chief of Pediatric Pulmonology
Department of Pediatrics
New York Methodist Hospital

Sonu Sahni, MD
Clinical Researcher
Department of Pulmonary, Critical Care and Sleep Medicine
North Shore-LIJ Health System

Rakesh Shah, **MD**, **FCCP**
Chief of Thoracic Radiology
Departments of Radiology and Medicine
North Shore University Hospital
Associate Professor of Radiology
Hofstra North Shore-LIJ School of Medicine

Abhishek Sharma, **MD**
Fellow, Division of Cardiology
SUNY Downstate Medical Center

Susan Smith, **ANP-C**
Department of Pulmonary, Sleep and Critical Care Medicine
ProHealth Care Associates

TABLES

FIGURES

Introduction

Pulmonary hypertension (PH) was only recently thought to describe a relatively rare but quickly fatal disease classically affecting young women. We now know PH is a problem which complicates a wide variety of medical illnesses, from genetically based sickle and Gauchers disease, to millions of individuals with COPD and congestive heart failure. It may complicate pulmonary embolism following surgery and many critical illnesses such as acute respiratory distress syndrome (ARDS). Because it is so pervasive, it is imperative that physicians across medical and surgical specialties and subspecialties have in-depth knowledge of diagnosis and management.

PH is now embedded as a key part of pulmonary, cardiology, and rheumatologic practice. Primary care physicians need to have good working knowledge to permit early recognition of PH. Treatment now permits stabilization and even regression of many of the pathologic components of PH utilizing available phosphodiesterase inhibitors, endothelin receptor antagonists, and prostacyclin-derived therapies. Many new and innovative treatment options are on the near horizon in various stages of development.

This handbook aims at providing a comprehensive, but concise, summary of the major diagnostic and therapeutic components of PH. It seeks to provide a useful practical framework of information relevant to primary care and specialist physicians as well as other health care providers involved with the diagnosis and treatment of this emerging public health problem.

1

Definitions and Classification

by Alan Fein, MD

The definition of pulmonary hypertension (PH) has evolved gradually over the seventy-plus years since pulmonary artery pressure (PAP) was first measured. Part of the challenge in defining normal from abnormal PAP occurred due to the need for right heart catheterization to obtain accurate measurements and the paucity of patients with severe PH. During that time, a series of international conferences have been convened by the World Health Organization (WHO) to gather experts in the field to debate the best definition and classification of the pulmonary hypertensive diseases. These meetings have generally been successful at developing a working definition and classification system that have gained widespread acceptance and is broadly used throughout the field today.

PH is currently defined as a mean PAP (mPAP) >25 mm Hg in the absence of elevated pulmonary venous pressure usually defined as a pulmonary capillary wedge pressure (PCWP), left atrial pressure (LAP), or left ventricular end-diastolic pressure (LVEDP) ≤15 mm Hg. The rationale of this definition is based on the idea that mPAP in normal individuals is about 14 mm Hg with a standard deviation of 3.3 mm Hg. Thus, a mPAP >2 standard deviations above the mean would be about 21 mm Hg. An mPAP of 21-24 falls into a borderline category that may be considered by some as early or mild PH. However, mean PAP increases with age and with elevation of pulmonary venous pressure, such that older individuals and patients with borderline elevation of LVEDP may approach 21-24 mm Hg and still be within 2 standard deviations of normal. In addition to mPAP >25 mm Hg, an increase in pulmonary vascular resistance (PVR) above 3 Woods units is often included in the definition of PH.

There has been disagreement regarding whether patients who have an mPAP <25 mm Hg at rest but who demonstrate an increase in mPAP above a certain threshold during exercise should be considered to have PH. At one time, an increase in mPAP >30 mm Hg during exercise was defined as exercise-induced PH. However, the increase in mPAP during exercise is very much dependent on the increase in cardiac output and considerable variation in the change in mPAP during exercise exists between individuals, making it difficult to identify at what point a pulmonary hypertensive response to exercise is present. As a result, changes in mPAP during exercise were dropped from the definition of PH at the most recent WHO symposium.

Most cases of PH result from an increase in pulmonary vascular tone and to a greater extent pulmonary vascular remodeling that is characterized by endothelial cell proliferation, medial hypertrophy, and thrombosis, and may reflect an imbalance between local vasodilators such as nitric oxide and prostacyclin, and vasoconstrictors such as thromboxane and endothelin-1. The mPAP at which symptoms of PH develop varies significantly, depending on comorbid illness and age. However, rising pressures over time may presage significant symptomatic disease associated with dyspnea, exercise limitation, and if not controlled, the development of right ventricle failure.

While the PH syndrome had been recognized for centuries, formal classification did not start until the 1970s when the WHO organized the first international meeting on PH. The first well-characterized case of PH reported in 1984 referred to the condition as "pulmonary sclerosis." Little changed from that initial report until 1954 when Dreysdale reported a series of patients with PH who had abnormal pulmonary vascular remodeling. He referred to these cases as "primary pulmonary hypertension" to signify that the cause of the elevated PAP was due to a "primary" defect in the pulmonary circulation rather than arising "secondary" to abnormalities of hypoxia, elevated pulmonary venous pressure, or other disease proccesses. At the first WHO meeting on PH, a distinction was made between primary and secondary PH, and primary PH was divided into the "arterial plexiform," "veno-occlusive," and "thromboembolic" forms.[3] At the next conference in 1998, causes of PH that were due to other medical conditions were discussed. However, the terms "primary" and "secondary" became confusing. For example, patients with PH associated with scleroderma were described as have "secondary" pulmonary hypertension when they had a disease that pathologically was very similar to primary pulmonary hypertension.[4]

At the third World Symposium on Pulmonary Arterial Hypertension in 2003, a new classification system was proposed that was based on new understandings of disease mechanisms. This classification system proposed five groups of pulmonary hypertensive disease. This five-group classification was further modified at the fourth WHO meeting at Dana Point, CA, in 2008 and again recently at the fifth WHO symposium in Nice, France, in 2013 (**Table 1.1**). The current classification system has sought to rationalize the multiplicity of causes, attempting to group conditions based on our current understanding of pathophysiology.[2] This process begins to provide a focus for clinical approaches based on the diverse pathobiologies of PH.

The Dana Point classification proffered in 2008 and endorsed by the WHO identifies five broad categories. This schema takes into account the uncertain understanding of the pathologies and the recognition that some PH may be multifactorial with many underlying processes acting in concert to elevate pulmonary pressures. Outcomes in the many types and iterations of PH may be quite different, requiring individualized strategic approaches.

TABLE 1.1 — Classification of Pulmonary Hypertension

1. Pulmonary arterial hypertension (PAH)
    1.1 Idiopathic PAH
    1.2 Heritable PAH
        1.2.1 BMPR2
        1.2.2 ALK-1, ENG, SMAD9, CAV1, KCNK3
        1.2.3 Unknown
    1.3 Drug- and toxin-induced
    1.4 Associated with:
        1.4.1 Connective tissue disease
        1.4.2 HIV infection
        1.4.3 Portal hypertension
        1.4.4 Congenital heart diseases
        1.4.5 Schistosomiasis
1'. Pulmonary veno-occlusive disease (PVOD) and/or pulmonary capillary hemangiomatosis (PCH)
1''. Persistent pulmonary hypertension of the newborn (PPHN)
2. Pulmonary hypertension due to left heart disease
    2.1 Left ventricular systolic dysfunction
    2.2 Left ventricular diastolic dysfunction
    2.3 Valvular disease
    2.4 Congenital/acquired left heart inflow/outflow tract obstruction and congenital cardiomyopathies
3. Pulmonary hypertension due to lung diseases and/or hypoxia
    3.1 Chronic obstructive pulmonary disease
    3.2 Interstitial lung disease
    3.3 Other pulmonary diseases with mixed restrictive and obstructive pattern
    3.4 Sleep-disordered breathing
    3.5 Alveolar hypoventilation disorders
    3.6 Chronic exposure to high altitude
    3.7 Developmental lung diseases
4. Chronic thromboembolic pulmonary hypertension (CTEPH)

Continued

TABLE 1.1 — *Continued*

5. Pulmonary hypertension with unclear multifactorial mechanisms
    5.1 Hematologic disorders: chronic hemolytic anemia, myeloproliferative disorders, splenectomy
    5.2 Systemic disorders: sarcoidosis, pulmonary Langerhans cell and histiocytosis, lymphangioleiomyomatosis
    5.3 Metabolic disorders: glycogen storage disease, Gaucher disease, thyroid disorders
    5.4 Others: tumoral obstruction, fibrosing mediastinitis, chronic renal failure, segmental PH

Adapted from Simonneau G, et al. *J Am Coll Cardiol*. 2013;62(25 suppl):D34-D41.

Group 1

This group, termed PAH, includes all PH diseases that are caused by abnormal increases in pulmonary vascular tone and remodeling and include five subgroups:

- Group 1.1: Idiopathic PAH (formerly known as primary pulmonary hypertension)
- Group 1.2: Heritable PH
- Group 1.3: Drug-induced PAH
- Group 1.4: Associated PAH (APAH) referring to PAH associated with one of five diseases
- Group 1': Pulmonary veno-occlusive disease and pulmonary capillary hemangiomatosis— two rare diseases characterized by obliterative lesions in the pulmonary venules or capillaries rather than in the distal pulmonary arteries as is seen in PAH.

PAH is almost always a progressive form of PH that leads to severe elevation in mPAP and right heart failure. The average mPAP in large registries of PAH ranges from 52-55 mm Hg, well above the threshold of 25 mm Hg that defines PH and well above the mPAP that is encounter in Group 2 and 3 PH associated with chronic heart and lung disease.

The heritable forms of PAH include mutations in the gene for bone morphogenic protein receptor-2 (BMPR2), which is the best characterized genetic defect associated with PAH. Mutations in BMPR2 have also been reported in up to 20% of patients with idiopathic pulmonary arterial hypertension (IPAH) as well. Other mutations, including those in alkaline kinase-like 1 (ALK-1) and endoglin that are closely related to BMPR2, have also been reported as well as seemingly unrelated mutations in the potassium channel (KRV).

Drug-induced PH has been linked to the prior use of fenfluramine/phentermine phentolamine in weight-loss therapy. Outbreaks of PAH associated with the use of aminorex in Europe during the 1970s and again with fenfluramine/phentermine referred to as fen-phen in the 1990s led to the removal of these diet pills from the market. SSRIs have been associated with PH in the newborn when taken by mothers in early trimesters. Causation mechanisms need to be elucidated in many of the toxin-associated PAH syndromes, including cocaine, chemotherapeutic agents, and amphetamines.

Connective tissue disease, itself a heterogeneous category, is commonly associated with PAH, particularly in the limited cutaneous form of scleroderma, where PAH has been reported in approximately 10% of cases.[4] In systemic sclerosis, PH may be multifactorial including PAH or PH associated with left ventricular diastolic dysfunction and/or interstitial fibrosis. Many connective tissue and rheumatologic illnesses, such as SLE, rheumatoid arthritis (RA), and mixed connective tissue disease, are associated with pulmonary vascular disease and PH. The incidence of PAH in these latter conditions is less well studied than in systemic sclerosis.

Portal hypertension is often associated with PAH and has been related to the severity of cirrhosis. Approximately 2% to 3% of patient with portal hypertension and liver cirrhosis develop PAH. Frequently,

PVR is only mildly increased because of the associated increase in cardiac output. PAH is also seen in about 0.5% of patients with HIV infection, but the cause of the association is not understood.

Congenital heart diseases that result in significant left to right shunting is associated with PAH.[5] It is most commonly associated with Eisenmenger syndrome in which the increased pulmonary arterial flow caused by a left to right intracardiac shunt leads to pulmonary vascular remodeling and increased PVR. As PAP gradually rises, flow across the cardiac defect reverses and becomes more right to left causing hypoxia. This may occur at any time during development or late into adult life. A wide variety of congenital heart diseases may result in PAH with variable incidence (**Table 1.2** and **Table 1.3**). Included in this group are atrial and ventricular septal defects. Many are not fully reversible despite corrective surgery.

PAH associated with schistosomiasis is classified in Group 1 since presentation and natural history share similar characteristics with IPAH. While this group of parasites is common in Asia, Africa, and the Middle East, the incidence of significant complicating PAH is unknown. Obstruction by embolized eggs and secondary fibrosis is thought to be causative but treatment response is not well understood.

Finally, pulmonary veno-occlusive disease and pulmonary hemangiomatosis are rare causes of PAH. In these conditions, the pathophysiology is not fully understood and preliminary data indicates less responsiveness to standard therapy. While veno-occlusive disease shares some characteristics with more common varieties of PAH, presentation is characterized by rales on physical examination and pulmonary infiltrates on chest x-ray.

Regardless of the underlying etiology, the severity of PH patients with Group 1 PAH is usually classified by their functional capacity using a modification of the New York Heart Association's functional classification of heart failure (**Table 1.4**). Higher functional class is

TABLE 1.2 — Anatomic Classification of Congenital Systemic-to-Pulmonary Shunts Associated With PAH

1. Type
   - 1.1 Simple pre-tricuspid shunts
     - 1.1.1 Atrial septal defect (ASD)
       - 1.1.1.1 Ostium secundum
       - 1.1.1.2 Sinus venosus
       - 1.1.1.3 Ostium primum
     - 1.1.2 Total or partial unobstructed anomalous pulmonary venous return
   - 1.2 Simple post-tricuspid shunts
     - 1.2.1 Ventricular septal defect (VSD)
     - 1.2.2 Patent ductus arteriosus (PDA)
   - 1.3 Combined shunts (describe combination and define predominant defect)
   - 1.4 Complex congenital heart disease
     - 1.4.1 Complete atrioventricular septal defect
     - 1.4.2 Truncus arteriosus
     - 1.4.3 Single ventricle physiology with unobstructed pulmonary blood flow
     - 1.4.4 Transposition of the great arteries with VSD (without pulmonary stenosis) and/or PDA
     - 1.4.5 Other
2. Dimension (specify for each defect if >1)
   - 2.1 Hemodynamic (specify ratio of pulmonary-to-systemic blood flow)
     - 2.1.1 Restrictive (pressure gradient across the defect)
     - 2.1.2 Nonrestrictive
   - 2.2 Anatomic
     - 2.2.1 Small to moderate (ASD ≤2.0 cm and VSD ≤1.0 cm)
     - 2.2.2 Large (ASD >2.0 cm and VSD >1.0 cm)
3. Direction of shunt
   - 3.1 Predominantly systemic-to-pulmonary
   - 3.2 Predominantly pulmonary-to-systemic
   - 3.3 Bidirectional
4. Associated cardiac and extracardiac abnormalities
5. Repair status
   - 5.1 Unoperated
   - 5.2 Palliated (specify type of operation[s], age at surgery)
   - 5.3 Repaired (specify type of operation[s], age at surgery)

Adapted from Simonneau G, et al. *J Am Coll Cardiol*. 2009;54(suppl 1):S43-S54.

TABLE 1.3 — Clinical Classification of Congenital Systemic-to-Pulmonary Shunts Associated With PAH

A	Eisenmenger syndrome	Patients with unrepaired systemic-to-pulmonary shunts resulting from large, nonrestrictive defects leading to a severe, progressive increase in pulmonary vascular resistance, bidirectional shunting, and ultimately reversed shunting with central cyanosis
B	PAH with moderate to large defects	Pulmonary vascular resistance is mildly to moderately increased, systemic-to-pulmonary shunt is still present, and no cyanosis is present at rest
C	PAH with small defects	Smaller defects generally include ventricular septal defect ≤1 cm and atrial septal defect ≤2 cm, and clinical picture is similar to idiopathic PAH
D	PAH following corrective cardiac surgery	CHD has been corrected, but PAH is present either immediately after surgery or recurs several months or years after surgery in the absence of significant residual shunts

Adapted from Simonneau G, et al. *J Am Coll Cardiol*. 2009;54(suppl 1):S43-S54.

associated with worse prognosis and indicates the need for more aggressive medical therapy (see *Chapter 5*).

Group 2

PH related to left heart disease is the most commonly encountered form of PH in clinical practice.[7] Left ventricular systolic dysfunction, diastolic dysfunction, or valvular disease can result in elevated left-sided filling pressure that raises pulmonary venous pressure.

TABLE 1.4 — Functional Classifications of Pulmonary Hypertension

Class I	Patients with pulmonary hypertension but without resulting limitation of physical activity. Ordinary physical activity does not cause undue dyspnea or fatigue, chest pain, or near syncope.
Class II	Patients with pulmonary hypertension resulting in slight limitation of physical activity. They are comfortable at rest. Ordinary physical activity causes undue dyspnea or fatigue, chest pain, or near syncope.
Class III	Patients with pulmonary hypertension resulting in marked limitation of physical activity. They are comfortable at rest. Less-than-ordinary physical activity causes undue dyspnea or fatigue, chest pain, or near syncope.
Class IV	Patients with pulmonary hypertension with inability to carry out any physical activity without symptoms. These patients manifest signs of right heart failure. Dyspnea and/or fatigue may even be present at rest. Discomfort is increased by any physical activity.

Normally the transpulmonary gradient (TPG), which is the difference between mPAP and LVEDP, is no more than 12 mm Hg. As LVEDP rises above 15 mm Hg, mPAP can approach or exceed the 25 mm Hg (the threshold that defines PH) despite a normal TPG. As a result, PH commonly complicates cardiomyopathy and mitral and/or aortic valve disease.

PVR is often within normal limits (3 Woods units) because the TPG remains normal. In some instances, however, PVR is elevated and the TPG is increased.

In these instances, PH is progressive and may have clinical similarity to Group 1 patients. One hypothesis is that TPG is elevated in these patients due to an increase in pulmonary vascular tone that is meant to retard blood flow through the lung to decrease left-sided filling pressures. In fact, treatment of Group 2 PH with pulmonary vasodilators when the TPG is elevated can result in further elevation of pulmonary venous pressure and the development of pulmonary edema. It should be emphasized that the natural history and treatment response to available PAH-directed therapies in patients with Group 2 PH and elevated TPG are not well studied and that available PH therapies are not FDA approved in this category.

Group 3

Chronic lung disease or exposure to an oxygen-poor environment constitutes the second most common cause of PH. Any significant pulmonary disease, either restrictive or obstructive, may be associated with PH. Reduced oxygen tension and respiratory acidosis increase pulmonary vascular tone and contribute to pulmonary vascular remodeling. Loss of pulmonary vessels occurs in emphysema, pulmonary fibrosis, and other structural lung diseases, and contributes to the increase in PVR. Common causes of Group 3 patients include COPD, interstitial lung disease, sleep disordered breathing and hypoventilation, and other mixed obstructive and restrictive lung diseases.

COPD is frequently associated with mild to moderate PH, although elevation of mPAP >30-35 mm Hg is unusual. In the rare instances where PAP is significantly higher, it is referred to as out of proportion PH and may reflect primary pulmonary vascular disease.[9] This has been demonstrated in approximately 2% of patients in COPD in studies in which right heart catheterization was performed. This pattern has been associated with severely reduced diffusing capacity on pulmonary function testing.[10] Issues related to out of proportion PH in this group are significant. Separating Group 3 PH from patients with Group 1 PAH and chronic lung disease often becomes a matter of clinical judgment.

The association of PH with obstructive sleep apnea is strong but the etiologic basis is less certain. Risk increases when OSA is associated with obesity hypoventilation syndrome and in many cases patients will have Group 2 PH owing to LV diastolic dysfunction. Patients with developmental lung disease may also have Group 3 PH, particularly if their disease is associated with chronic hypoxemia or hypercapnia. Group 3 PH is also common in populations who live at high altitude, usually in excess of 3000 m, and has been linked to a variety of genetic factors that may predispose patients to the development of PH.

Group 4

Chronic thromboembolic pulmonary hypertension (CTEPH) results from the obstruction and subsequent fibrosis of the pulmonary vascular bed following incomplete resolution of acute or recurrent PE (see *Chapter 13*).[11] The development of CTEPH has been reported in up to 4% of patients following acute PE, but many patients with CTEPH have no known history of PE. Thus, it is likely that CTEPH is more common in PE than has been reported. Persistent obstruction to the pulmonary vascular bed increases PVR and eventually results in right heart failure.

The mechanisms inhibiting resolution of the initial embolic episode are not well known but may reflect failure of thrombolysis and persistent inflammation limiting remodeling of the endothelial bed. Increased circulating factor 8 and antiphospholipid antibodies has been observed in up to 20% of CTEPH. Alternatively, no consistent association with protein S or C deficiency has been demonstrated. It has been suggested that rather than always being the result of recurrent and or nonresolving PE, CTEPH is the result of a primary arteriopathy with repetitive in situ thrombosis.

Pulmonary vascular remodeling has also been observed in pulmonary vessels that are free of emboli or thrombosis suggesting that increased blood flow through nonaffected vessels results in pulmonary vascular disease that contributes to CTEPH. CTEPH was initially categorized as either proximal or distal, depending on the site of obstruction and how amenable it is to surgical thromboendarterectomy. The distinction between Group 1 and Group 4 PH is important because the later requires long-term anticoagulation and may be amenable to pulmonary endarterectomy that can result in marked improvements in pulmonary hemodynamics and functional status.

Group 5

This is a group which encompasses a wide variety of diseases and syndromes in which PH is the result of multiple mechanisms and/or etiologies for which the mechanism of disease is unclear. Included are such diverse conditions as myeloproliferative disorders and sarcoidosis. PH is increasingly recognized in sarcoidosis and may result from destruction of the pulmonary vascular bed by parenchymal fibrosis.[12] While usually a manifestation of severe sarcoidosis, even patients with minimal disease may be affected. PH is associated with the severity of pulmonary functional impairment, particularly with low diffusing capacity and exercise desaturation.

Other causes of PAH include a variety of hemolytic anemia, most commonly, sickle cell disease. In these cases, rates of clinically significant PAH approach 25%.[6] Most of these cases are associated with increased cardiac output due to chronic anemia and/or elevated left-sided filling pressures, but an increased TPG in the setting of normal LVEDP has been reported in approximately 6% of patients with sickle cell disease. Current prevailing theory about causation is that recurrent in situ microthrombosis and nitric oxide consumption by hemolyzing cells may contribute to pulmonary vasoconstriction and fibrosis. The natural history and response to therapeutic interventions in PH associated with sickle cell disease remains an area of active investigation. Present treatment goals focus on management of the underlying anemia and the judicious use of pulmonary vasodilators in selected patients.[6]

Other processes rarely associated with PH include lymphangiomyomatosis, pulmonary histiocytosis, and vasculitis. Glycogen storage disorders such as Gaucher's disease may lead to PH when glucocerebroside accumulates in the lung parenchymal.[13] Thyroid disease, including hypothyroidism and autoimmune thyroiditis, have also been associated with PH. Tumor emboli and chronic renal failure requiring hemodialysis may also develop PH.

Key Points

- PH is defined as a mPAP >25 mm Hg in the absence of left-sided filling pressure ≥15 mm Hg. In the great majority of patients, PVR exceeds 3 Woods units.
- PH is categorized into five groups that include:
  – PAH
  – PH owing to left heart disease
  – PH owing to chronic lung disease
  – Chronic thromboembolic pulmonary hypertension
  – PH with multifactorial unclear mechanisms.
- Group 1 PAH is the most severe and least common cause of PH. The most common causes of PH are left-sided heart disease and chronic lung disease.
- CTEPH occurs in approximately 4% of patients with acute PE, but many patients with CTEPH are unaware of any history of DVT or PE. CTEPH should be excluded in all patients with PH because its prognosis and management differ substantially from Group 1 PAH.

- With the exception of one medication that has recently been approved for the treatment of CTEPH, all medications currently approved for the treatment of PH are indicated for Group 1 PAH only. **1**

REFERENCES

1. Houtchens J, Martin D, Klinger JR. Diagnosis and management of pulmonary arterial hypertension. *Pulm Med.* 2011;2011:845864.

2. Simonneau G, Gatzoulis MA, Adatia I, et al. Updated clinical classification of pulmonary hypertension. *J Am Coll Cardiol.* 2013;62(25 suppl):D34-D41.

3. Deng Z, Morse JH, Slager SL, et al. Familial primary pulmonary hypertension (gene PPH1) is caused by mutations in the bone morphogenetic protein receptor-II gene. *Am J Hum Genet.* 2000;67(3):737-744.

4. Kawut SM, Taichman DB, Archer-Chicko CL, Palevsky HI, Kimmel SE. Hemodynamics and survival in patients with pulmonary arterial hypertension related to systemic sclerosis. *Chest.* 2003;123(2):344-350.

5. Rose ML, Strange G, King I, et al. Congenital heart disease-associated pulmonary arterial hypertension: preliminary results from a novel registry. *Intern Med J.* 2012;42(8):874-879.

6. Gladwin MT, Sachdev V, Jison ML, et al. Pulmonary hypertension as a risk factor for death in patients with sickle cell disease. *N Engl J Med.* 2004;350(9):886-895.

7. Lam CS, Roger VL, Rodeheffer RJ, Borlaug BA, Enders FT, Redfield MM. Pulmonary hypertension in heart failure with preserved ejection fraction: a community-based study. *J Am Coll Cardiol.* 2009;53(13):1119-1126.

8. Seeger W, Adir Y, Barberà JA, et al. Pulmonary hypertension in chronic lung diseases. *J Am Coll Cardiol.* 2013;62(25 Suppl):D109-D116.

9. Hoeper MM, Andreas S, Bastian A, et al. Pulmonary hypertension due to chronic lung disease: updated Recommendations of the Cologne Consensus Conference 2011. *Int J Cardiol.* 2011; 154 Suppl 1:S45-S53.

10. Chaouat A, Bugnet AS, Kadaoui N, et al. Severe pulmonary hypertension and chronic obstructive pulmonary disease. *Am J Respir Crit Care Med.* 2005;172(2):189-194.

11. Pengo V, Lensing AW, Prins MH, et al; Thromboembolic Pulmonary Hypertension Study Group. Incidence of chronic thromboembolic pulmonary hypertension after pulmonary embolism. *N Engl J Med*. 2004;350(22):2257-2264.

12. Handa T, Nagai S, Miki S, et al. Incidence of pulmonary hypertension and its clinical relevance in patients with sarcoidosis. *Chest*. 2006;129(5):1246-1252.

13. Lo SM, Liu J, Chen F, et al. Pulmonary vascular disease in Gaucher disease: clinical spectrum, determinants of phenotype and long-term outcomes of therapy. *J Inherit Metab Dis*. 2011;34(3):643-650.

2

Practical Epidemiology and Clinical Presentation

by Alan Fein, MD

General Considerations

The approach to patients with pulmonary hypertension (PH) requires understanding of clinical presentation, natural history, and risk factors. Patients with PH may present with symptoms of increasing dyspnea and disability or may arrive to the clinician with only abnormal findings on diagnostic tests in the absence of significant symptoms. Textbook presentations of pulmonary arterial hypertension (PAH) are, unfortunately, not the normal. Multifactorial PH is more often the rule rather than the exception. For example, significant PH is increasingly recognized in the elderly patient presenting with dyspnea but is usually caused by chronic heart or lung disease.

Since PH-specific medications are indicated only for WHO Group 1 PAH (see *Chapter 1* for definitions and classifications), it is important to differentiate the clinical phenotypes of PH so that appropriate therapy is initiated. Recently, it has been suggested that PH be reclassified based on demographic and hemodynamic variables, and potentially, the presence of certain biomarkers.[1] It is incumbent on physicians managing patients with PH to recognize not only the presence of PH, but also the natural history of the many PH phenotypes in order to effectively guide a program of treatment.

Epidemiology

Our understanding of the epidemiology of PH continues to evolve. As classification has become more sophisticated and accurate, the ability of epidemiologists to understand causation and natural history has significantly improved (**Figure 2.1**). This trend has resulted in improved knowledge of the presentation and progression of PAH since its original description in the late 19th century when both "sclerosis" of pulmonary arteries and consequent "cyanosis" were recognized as prominent features. PAH was further characterized following the advent of cardiac catheterization when elevated mPAP and pulmonary vascular resistance (PVR) were identified as important features of PAH.

FIGURE 2.1 — Natural History of Pulmonary Hypertension

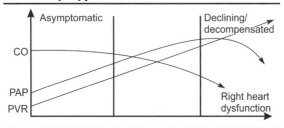

Physiologic changes of pulmonary hypertension. With progressive increase in PVR, the PAP initially increases until a failing right heart can no longer generate the required pressures to maintain cardiac output.

Adapted from Friedman EB, et al. In: Mandel J, Taichman DB, eds. *Pulmonary Vascular Disease*. Philadelphia, PA: Elsevier; 2006.

Presently, the natural history of PAH is felt to be a disease process that slowly obliterates or narrows the pulmonary vascular bed causing a progressive rise in pulmonary vascular resistance (PVR). Initially, the right ventricle responds by increasing pulmonary arterial pressure (PAP) to maintain cardiac output, but eventually the rise in PVR becomes too great, the right ventricle begins to fail, and PAP falls. This final phase of the disease results in decompensated right heart failure and death from cardiogenic shock (**Figure 2.1**).

Much of the epidemiology of PAH has been derived from a series of large case registries. A National Institute of Health database compiled in the 1980s was one of the first registries to describe the characteristics of PAH, which at that time was more commonly referred to as primary PH.[2] While PAH was found to be rare, with incidence reported over a wide range from 1 to 50 per million population, it resulted in >200,000 hospitalizations/year by the 21st century. Generally associated features included young age (mean age 36 ± 15 years), higher prevalence in women (63%), the presence of Raynaud's symptoms, and rapid progression to death within 3 years of diagnosis (median survival 2.8 years). Although most patients were deemed "primary" or "idiopathic," some reported a family history of PAH or the use of anorectic amphetamine derivatives for diet control.

More recent databases including those reported by the French National Registry and the US-based Registry to Evaluate Early and Long-Term PAH Management (REVEAL) demonstrate a greater proportion of female patients and older age (mean age $50\text{-}52 \pm 15$ years).[3,4]

Two distinct subtypes of PAH have been identified based on the patient's age. Older patients (>50 years of age) appear to have more delayed diagnosis and are more likely to have comorbid medical illnesses, which can make the diagnosis of PAH more challenging. Included in these comorbid illnesses are hypertension, diabetes, coronary artery disease, and obesity patients with multifactorial cardiac risk factors such as diabetes, hyperlipidemia, and obstructive sleep apnea, frequently known as the metabolic syndrome, also appear to be at increased risk of right ventricular dysfunction and enlargement.

Left ventricular diastolic dysfunction plays a significant role in PH, particularly in older patients with associated coronary artery disease and diabetes, and needs to be distinguished. Stiff and fibrotic ventricles result in elevated pulmonary venous pressures, especially during exercise. The pulmonary capillary wedge pressure (PCWP) estimates, but does not always accurately measure, the left ventricular end-diastolic pressure (LVEDP). Edema was described more frequently in these older patients, while syncope and near syncope were more common in younger patients. Despite less severe hemodynamic impairment in the older group, prognosis was significantly worse.

The dismal survival initially reported in PH seems to be significantly improving; this has been hypothesized to be the result of the introduction of PAH-specific therapy over the past decade.

Risk Assessment

It is clear that many patients currently classified within the same categories may have variable prognosis based on differences in underlying prognosis. For example, PAH associated with connective tissue disease and PAH associated with congenital heart disease are both included in WHO Group 1, although long-term survival is considerably better in PAH related to congenital heart disease.[5] Original databases utilizing incident rather than prevalent cases may have negatively skewed the interpretation of outcomes.[4,10] Over the past 3 decades, survival in IPAH has improved from approximately 50% at 3 years[2] to 65% at 5 years[3,4] (**Figure 2.2**). Factors associated with poor outcome include male sex, high right atrial pressure, and low cardiac output. Renal disease, exercise performance, supplementary oxygen dependence, and older age (**Figure 2.3**) also adversely affect outcome.[4,6] In a recent prospective study of patients with PAH associated with systemic sclerosis, survival was 80%, 78%, and 56% at 1-, 2-, and 3-year follow-up periods, respectively.[12]

The REVEAL risk calculator is one of several risk assessment tools that can be used to predict survival in PAH using data derived from analysis of national PAH databases. The REVEAL risk calculator uses many of

FIGURE 2.2 — Observed vs Predicted Survival in Patients With Pulmonary Hypertension

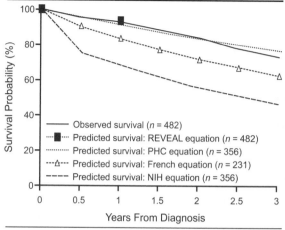

Ling Y, et al. *Am J Respir Crit Care Med*. 2012;186(8):790-796.

the same variables employed in the prediction formulas of other databases but gives them somewhat different weight (**Figure 2.4**).

Heritability, Genetics, and Environmental Factors

Up to 10% of patients with PH have a family history of PH. There appears to be approximately a 10% chance of developing PH in first-order relatives of incident cases. At the turn of the century, a mutation in the gene that encodes the bone morphogenic protein type 2 receptor (BMPR2) was identified in several large cohorts of familial pulmonary hypertension. Mutations of BMPR2 are the most commonly associated genetic defect associated with PAH. BMPR2 mutations have been reported in up to 75% of familial PAH cases and up to 25% of sporadic cases of IPAH as well.[7] Over 300 mutations of BMPR2 have been identified in association with PAH. Interestingly, none of these

FIGURE 2.3 — Survival in Pulmonary Hypertension, Age

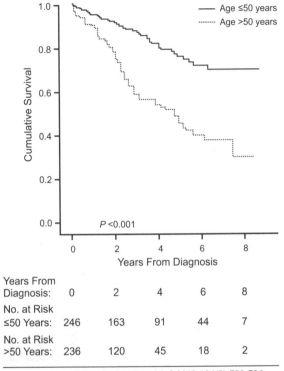

Years From Diagnosis:	0	2	4	6	8
No. at Risk ≤50 Years:	246	163	91	44	7
No. at Risk >50 Years:	236	120	45	18	2

Ling Y, et al. *Am J Respir Crit Care Med.* 2012;186(8):790-796.

has been found to be associated with PAH associated with connective tissue disease, HIV infection, or portal hypertension.

Other mutations associated with PAH include activin A receptor type II-like 1 (ACVRL1) and endoglin. The latter is seen in PAH associated with hereditary hemorrhagic telangiectasia. All three of these mutations occur in members of the transforming growth factor (TGF-β) superfamily of receptors, which modulate normal vascular development. Other less commonly identified mutations that have been associated with PAH include CAV1, the gene that encodes for a membrane protein of caveolae, and KCNK3, the gene that encodes the pH- and hypoxia-sensitive potassium channel in the 2-pore domain superfamily.

Low genetic penetrance is another characteristic of heritable PH. Approximately one in eight carriers of the BMPR2 mutations will develop PAH, suggesting that environmental factors may be interacting with genetic predisposition to cause clinical disease. Patients with heritable pulmonary arterial hypertension (HPAH) manifest their disease at an earlier age than patients with IPAH and tend to have more severe disease as evidenced by higher PVR and lower cardiac output at diagnosis, less responsiveness to pulmonary vasodilators, and greater risk of progression to lung transplant or death.

■ Drug and Toxin-Related PAH

In the 1960s, the use of appetite suppressants resulted in a significant increase in recognized PAH (odds ratio [OR] to >50-fold).[8] The risk for developing PAH increases with duration of drug exposure beyond 3 months and the average interval between onset of drug use and development of PAH is around 4 years. It also appears that anorectic agents enhance the risk of PAH more in patients who are already predisposed to developing PAH, such as those with collagen vascular disease. PAH is likely to occur relatively quickly after starting these medications, usually within 2 years of initiation. In US registries, the mean age at the onset of PAH was 46 years and three quarters were women. The early age and female preponderance is similar to that seen in idiopathic PAH but may reflect the increased use of anorectic agents in this population.

The anorectic drugs, aminorex fumarate, fenfluramine, and dexfenfluramine, have been directly associated with a marked increase in the incidence of PAH, most likely due to their effect of increasing serotonin levels (**Table 2.1**). Epidemics of PAH associated with the use of these appetite suppressants first in Europe

FIGURE 2.4 — REVEAL Registry: PAH Risk Score Calculator

REVEAL	PAH Risk Score			
WHO Group Subgroup	APAH-CTD +1	APAH-PoPH +2	FPAH +2	☐
Demographics and Comorbidities	Renal Insufficiency +1		Males Age >60 yr +2	☐
NYHA/WHO Functional Class	I −2	III +1	IV +2	☐
Vital Signs	SBP <110 mm Hg +1		HR >92 BPM +1	☐
6MWD Test	≥440 m −1		<165 m +1	☐
BNP	<50 pg/mL −2		>180 pg/mL +1	☐
Echocardiogram	Pericardial Effusion +1			☐
Pulmonary Function Test	% Predicted DLCO ≥80 −1		% Predicted DLCO ≤32 +1	☐
Right Heart Catheterization	mRAP >20 mm Hg within 1 y +1		PVR >32 Wood units +2	☐

Sum of Above ☐

\+ **6**

= Risk Score ☐

Key: APAH, associated pulmonary arterial hypertension; BNP, brain natriuretic peptide; BPM, beats per minute; CTD, connective tissue disease; DLCO, diffusing capacity of lung for carbon monoxide; FPAH, familial pulmonary arterial hypertension; HR, heart rate; mRAP, mean right atrial pressure; NYHA, New York Heart Association; PAH, pulmonary
Continued

FIGURE 2.4 — *Continued*

arterial hypertension; PoPH, portopulmonary hypertension; PVR, pulmonary vascular resistance; REVEAL Registry, Registry to Evaluate Early and Long-term Pulmonary Arterial Hypertension Disease Management; SBP, systolic BP; WHO, World Health Organization.

2

If N-terminal proBNP is available and BNP is not, listed cut points are replaced with <300 pg/mL and >1500 pg/mL.

Predicted 1-year survival is 95% to 100% for a score of 1-7, 90% to 95% for a score of 8, 85% to 90% for a score of 9, 70% to 85% for a score of 10-11, and <70% for scores >12.

Benza RL, et al. *Chest.* 2012;141(2):354-362.

TABLE 2.1 — Drugs and Toxins Associated With PAH

Confirmed	Probable
• Aminorex • Fenfluramine • Dexfenfluramine • Toxic rapeseed oil • Dasatinib	• Amphetamines • l-Tryptophan • Interferon

and later in the United States led to their removal from the market. Monoamine oxidase (MAO) inhibitors and selective serotonin reuptake inhibitors (SSRIs) have also been suggested as risk factors for PAH, although the link between these drugs and PAH is less certain. Interestingly, the use of SSRIs in pregnancy has been associated with an increased risk of infant PH in the neonatal period. Amphetamines used by intravenous or inhaled routes are also considered likely causes of elevated PAPs. The risk of PAH with other stimulants such as cocaine and St. John's wort remain unproven. Concern has also been raised regarding reports of PAH associated with the use of interferon or the tyrosine kinase inhibitor dasatinib. Survival of drug-induced PAH has been thought to be similar to idiopathic PAH since the introduction of specific therapy.[9,10]

■ Connective Tissue Disease

The incidence of PAH associated with connective tissue disease varies considerably among the various subtypes of this disease. However, pulmonary arterial vascular disease occurs much more frequently in most types of connective tissue disease than in the general population. PAH is particularly prevalent in the limited form of cutaneous scleroderma and in the CREST variant.[11] In these patients, the prevalence of PAH has been reported to be as high as 10% to 30%. Pulmonary vascular disease occurs in systemic lupus erythematosus (SLE), as well as in rheumatoid arthritis, Sjögren's syndrome, and mixed connective tissue disease. The presence of PH in connective tissue disease adversely affects prognosis, particularly in scleroderma.[12] Classification may be challenging since connective tissue disease affects lung and cardiac parenchyma, and PH can be related to either elevated pulmonary venous hypertension or hypoxic pulmonary vasoconstriction or both, rather than a primary pulmonary vasculopathy.

■ PH and HIV

Patients infected with human immunodeficiency virus (HIV) have a greatly increased risk of developing PAH compared to the general population. Before the introduction of highly active antiretroviral therapy (HAART), the incidence of PAH in HIV was reported to be as high as 0.5%.[13] As better control of HIV has been achieved, the incidence appears to have declined. Additionally, initiation of HAART therapy may delay onset of associated PAH. Direct viral invasion of the pulmonary vasculature is not thought to be the primary cause of pulmonary vascular disease. Rather, HIV infection likely results in increased production of endothelial growth factors in response to circulating cytokines and other inflammatory mediators stimulated by viral proteins such as nef and gp120. Practically, the treatment approach has not been differentiated from other types of Group 1 disease. Prognosis of HIV-associated PAH has improved, and two thirds of patients will survive beyond 3 years. Higher cardiac output and CD4 counts are independent predictors of survival.

■ Portal Hypertension

Porto-pulmonary hypertension (PPH) occurs in patients with liver disease, usually in the presence of cirrhosis and elevated portal pressures. It has been reported in one in 2% to 3% of patients with advanced liver disease. The mean age of patients with PPH is 50 and there is an equal frequency in men and women.[14] Pulmonary vascular resistance (PVR) is often lower and cardiac output is higher than in other forms of PAH. The etiology of PPH is uncertain but may be due in part to elevated endogenous vascular mediators which bypass the liver and act downstream on the pulmonary circulation. PH may also be exacerbated by the increased flow secondary to higher cardiac output that occurs in chronic liver disease. Pathologic findings are similar to those seen in PAH; prognosis related to the severity of cirrhosis and confers a worse prognosis than in idiopathic cases of PAH, with a 1-year survival of <50%. Liver transplantation sometimes reverses the PAH in these patients but operative complications may increase the overall mortality, particularly in patients who have a mean PAP >35 mm Hg.

■ Chronic Hemoglobinopathies and Hemolytic Anemias

PH associated with the hemolytic anemias, particularly sickle cell disease, were once listed with the other forms of associated PAH in WHO Group 1. However, in the most recent WHO classification system, this type of PH has been moved to Group 5—PH of unknown or unclear etiology. PH is common in sickle cell disease and some forms of thalassemia,[15] but when carefully assessed by right heart catheterization (RHC), PH in these patients is more likely to be due to elevation in left-sided filling pressure or increased cardiac output with only mild or no elevation in PVR. PH is less common in hereditary spherocytosis and paroxysmal nocturnal hemoglobinuria. The cause of vasculopathy is unknown but reduced bioavailability of NO has been suggested based on the idea that hemoglobin released from lysed red blood cells may scavenge NO in the pulmonary microcirculation and from the observation that arginase, an enzyme that metabolizes L-arginine—the major substrate for endothelial NO synthase—is increased in patients with sickle cell disease.

Regardless of the etiology, PH in patients with sickle disease is associated with a significantly worse prognosis.[16] Markers of hemolysis, such as plasma arginase, confer greater risk of PH and mortality. Unfortunately, attempts to counteract the perceived NO deficiency in sickle cell PH with the phosphodiesterase inhibitor sildenafil were not successful, and management has been directed instead toward optimizing management of the underlying anemia.

■ Congenital Heart Disease

Both generalists and physicians who specialize in PH will increasingly encounter patients with PAH associated with congenital heart disease termed APAH-CHD (WHO Group 1.5.5). This is a heterogeneous group with a wide diversity of pathologies and natural histories. Both APAH-CHD and IPAH are categorized as Group 1 PAH based on similar histopathology. However, the initiating pathophysiology is clearly different. APAH-CHD is a consequence of left to right intra-cardiac shunt and subsequent vascular remodeling due to exposure of the pulmonary circulation to high pulmonary blood flow.[17] Interestingly, right ventricular function may be well maintained for prolonged periods in APAH-CHF despite mPAP that is elevated as severely as that seen in patients with IPAH. This may occur because the right ventricular is exposed to high PAP at a younger age when it is still developing and the slow increase in PAP may allow the right ventricle to better adapt to the increase in afterload. As a result, the prognosis is considerably better in APAH-CHD than in other forms of PAH. For example, 5-year survival is 90% in patients with Eisenmenger's syndrome.[18]

The role of increased pulmonary vascular tone in PH associated with left-sided valvular heart disease or diastolic dysfunction has been recognized for many years. In many cases, PA diastolic pressure (dPAP) is elevated out of proportion to the elevation in left-sided filling pressures with a dPAP-PCWP >5 mm Hg. These patients may be subtly distinct from other Group 2 patients where elevated PAP occurs in proportion to the rise in pulmonary venous pressure. It has not been established that currently available PAH-specific therapy is effective in this group of patients. Reduction of pulmonary vascular tone with PAH-specific medications in these patients may increase blood flow through the lungs and further increase pulmonary venous pressure leading to pulmonary congestion and edema. Hence, they should be used with caution if at all in these patients.

■ Pulmonary Veno-occlusive Disease

This rare cause of PH results from occlusion and fibrosis in the pulmonary venous system. This form of PH has been identified in <1% of all patients with PH. The incidence of PVOD may be increased in patients with HIV or collagen vascular disease, or in those who have received some forms of chemotherapy or who have siblings with PVOD. Clinical features that are atypical for PAH but may be seen in PVOD include rales, clubbing, and pleural effusions. Unlike the clear lung fields described in PAH, veno-occlusive disease may be associated with radiographic evidence of interstitial edema and the presence of Kerley B lines.[19]

■ Chronic Thromboembolic Pulmonary Hypertension (CTEPH)

CTEPH is a progressive PH syndrome thought to arise from overt pulmonary arterial thrombosis in which obstruction results from embolization from remote locations or in situ thrombosis facilitated by vasculopathy. As such, it may overlap clinically with PAH. It is hypothesized that in CTEPH, single or multiple emboli do not sufficiently resolve to allow normal pulmonary blood flow. Since a significant proportion of pulmonary emboli (PE) are not clinically recognized, it is not unexpected that up to one third of patients with CTEPH do not have clearly documented episodes of PE.

In a prospective study of acute embolism, PH was evident in 4% of patients at 3 years.[20] After 3 years, it is thought that CTEPH is unlikely to develop. Larger perfusion defects and higher initial PAPs are among the risk factors for persistent PAH. Other risk factors include malignancy, thyroid disease, elevated factor VIII, antiphospholipid antibodies, infected catheters, or shunts. Since the availability of both medical and surgical therapy for CTEPH exists, screening for CTEPH may be warranted in high-risk patients, including those with recurrent emboli or thrombophilias or patients with large defects or central emboli detected in the workup of thromboembolism.

Clinical Presentation of PAH

The most common symptom of PAH is dyspnea with exertion which is not only a common complaint, but one that is present in many other cardiopulmonary illnesses. Due to the rarity of PAH, this disease is often not included in the differential diagnosis of progressive dyspnea, but in those patients in whom no other cause of dyspnea is found, PAH needs to be considered. Patients often present late in the course of PH, because symptoms of dyspnea and fatigue are nonspecific and often dismissed as deconditioning or depression when the initial workup fails to find any abnormalities of lung function. The diagnosis of PH in the early stage requires a high level of suspicion and careful interpretation of findings on exam and diagnostic tests. In some instances, elevated PAP may be detected during echocardiography performed as part of evaluation or follow-up of other cardiac conditions. Some patients may be asymptomatic at the time that PAP is found to be elevated. Patients may also present with minimal symptoms but express manifestations of the underlying diseases such as Raynaud's syndrome, joint deformities, rheumatoid arthritis, HIV, or thromboembolism that are associated with a high risk of developing PAH.

The clinician must be alert to the possibility of PAH causing a variety of complaints. Dyspnea either with exertion or at rest is by far the most common complaint, but patients will also describe fatigue, exertional chest pain, lightheadedness, or in more advanced disease, frank syncope. When right heart failure develops, lower extremity edema and hepatic congestion may predominate. Patients with PH other than Group 1 PAH often have a multiplicity of findings which makes the diagnosis challenging, including symptoms of heart failure, chronic lung disease, sleep apnea, anemia, or venous thromboembolism (**Table 2.2**).

TABLE 2.2 — Clinical Manifestations of Pulmonary Hypertension

Symptom	Estimated Frequency (% Patients)
Dyspnea	60
Fatigue	19
Chest pain	17
Near syncope	5
Syncope	8
Leg edema	3
Palpitations	5

In early stages of disease, the physical examination may be entirely normal or there may be only subtle prominence of the pulmonic component of the second heart sound. As PAP increases, splitting of the second heart sound, jugular venous distention, and a systolic ejection murmur representing tricuspid regurgitation heard best over the left sternal border may be observed. Many of these findings are the result of right ventricular pressure and volume overload with dilation of the tricuspid annulus and tricuspid regurgitation. If permitted to progress to overt right heart failure, hepatomegaly, ascites, and progressive peripheral edema are evident on physical examination.[21]

By convention, patients with established PH are classified according to the WHO functional classification. This schema has been adopted from the New York Heart Association classification of heart failure and has been accepted for both clinical evaluation and treatment and for the purpose of enrollment and follow-up during clinical trials. WHO functional class is defined as I) no symptoms, II) dyspnea with normal activity, III) dyspnea with less than ordinary activity, and IV) dyspnea with any activity or while at rest. Current treatment guidelines recommend oral pulmonary vasodilator therapy for patients in functional class II or III and intravenous epoprostenol infusion for those in functional class IV. The goal of PAH therapy is to achieve functional class II or lower or to improve at least one functional class.

Key Points

- WHO Group 1 PAH is a rare disease that occurs more commonly in women and in patients with connective tissue disease, portal hypertension, pulmonary embolism, HIV infection, left to right intracardiac shunts, and exposure to amphetamine-based appetite suppressants.
- Heritable PH occurs in approximately 10% of patients, and the great majority of these cases are caused by mutations in the gene that encodes bone morphogenic protein receptor-2.
- The epidemiology of PAH has changed significantly since the initial NIH registry was published over 30 years ago.
- More recent databases suggest that patients diagnosed with PAH today are older, more likely to

be female, and to have more comorbidities than patients diagnosed with PAH in the 1980s.

- After accounting for the change in demographics, survival of PAH appears to have improved with the availability of PAH-specific medications.

2

REFERENCES

1. Dweik RA, Rounds S, Erzurum SC, et al; ATS Committee on Pulmonary Hypertension Phenotypes. An official American Thoracic Society Statement: pulmonary hypertension phenotypes. *Am J Respir Crit Care Med*. 2014;189(3):345-355.

2. D'Alonzo GE, Barst RJ, Ayres SM, et al. Survival in patients with primary pulmonary hypertension. Results from a national prospective registry. *Ann Intern Med*. 1991;115(5):343-349.

3. Benza RL, Miller DP, Barst RJ, Badesch DB, Frost AE, McGoon MD. An evaluation of long-term survival from time of diagnosis in pulmonary arterial hypertension from the REVEAL Registry. *Chest*. 2012;142(2):448-456.

4. Ling Y, Johnson MK, Kiely DG, et al. Changing demographics, epidemiology, and survival of incident pulmonary arterial hypertension: results from the pulmonary hypertension registry of the United Kingdom and Ireland. *Am J Respir Crit Care Med*. 2012;186(8):790-796.

5. Krishnan U, Rosenzweig EB. Pulmonary arterial hypertension associated with congenital heart disease. *Clin Chest Med*. 2013; 34(4):707-717.

6. Thenappan T, Ryan JJ, Archer SL. Evolving epidemiology of pulmonary arterial hypertension. *Am J Respir Crit Care Med*. 2012;186(8):707-709.

7. Deng Z, Morse JH, Slager SL,et al. Familial primary pulmonary hypertension (gene PPH1) is caused by mutations in the bone morphogenetic protein receptor-II gene. *Am J Hum Genet*. 2000;67(3):737-744.

8. Rich S, Rubin L, Walker AM, Schneeweiss S, Abenhaim L. Anorexigens and pulmonary hypertension in the United States: results from the surveillance of North American pulmonary hypertension. *Chest*. 2000;117(3):870-874.

9. Rich S, Shillington A, McLaughlin V. Comparison of survival in patients with pulmonary hypertension associated with fenfluramine to patients with primary pulmonary hypertension. *Am J Cardiol*. 2003;92(11):1366-1368.

10. Humbert M, Sitbon O, Yaïci A, et al; French Pulmonary Arterial Hypertension Network. Survival in incident and prevalent cohorts of patients with pulmonary arterial hypertension. *Eur Respir J*. 2010;36(3):549-555.

11. Mukerjee D, St George D, Coleiro B, et al. Prevalence and outcome in systemic sclerosis associated pulmonary arterial hypertension: application of a registry approach. *Ann Rheum Dis*. 2003;62(11):1088-1093.

12. Kawut SM, Taichman DB, Archer-Chicko CL, Palevsky HI, Kimmel SE. Hemodynamics and survival in patients with pulmonary arterial hypertension related to systemic sclerosis. *Chest*. 2003;123(2):344-350.

13. Sitbon O, Lascoux-Combe C, Delfraissy JF, et al. Prevalence of HIV-related pulmonary arterial hypertension in the current antiretroviral therapy era. *Am J Respir Crit Care Med*. 2008; 177(1):108-113.

14. Fritz JS, Fallon MB, Kawut SM. Pulmonary vascular complications of liver disease. *Am J Respir Crit Care Med*. 2013; 187(2):133-143.

15. Parent F, Bachir D, Inamo J, et al. A hemodynamic study of pulmonary hypertension in sickle cell disease. *N Engl J Med*. 2011;365(1):44-53.

16. Gladwin MT, Sachdev V, Jison ML, et al. Pulmonary hypertension as a risk factor for death in patients with sickle cell disease. *N Engl J Med*. 2004;350(9):886-895.

17. Durmowicz AG, Stenmark KR. Mechanisms of structural remodeling in chronic pulmonary hypertension. *Pediatr Rev*. 1999;20(11):e91-e102.

18. Haworth SG, Hislop AA. Treatment and survival in children with pulmonary arterial hypertension: the UK Pulmonary Hypertension Service for Children 2001-2006. *Heart*. 2009; 95(4):312-317.

19. Holcomb BW Jr, Loyd JE, Ely EW, Johnson J, Robbins IM. Pulmonary veno-occlusive disease: a case series and new observations. *Chest*. 2000;118(6):1671-1679.

20. Pengo V, Lensing AW, Prins MH, et al; Thromboembolic Pulmonary Hypertension Study Group. Incidence of chronic thromboembolic pulmonary hypertension after pulmonary embolism. *N Engl J Med*. 2004;350(22):2257-2264.

21. Mathier MA. Pulmonary hypertension owing to left heart disease. *Clin Chest Med*. 2013;34(4):683-694.

3 Diagnosis

by Abhishek Sharma, MD and
Jason M. Lazar, MD, MPH

Pulmonary hypertension (PH) is characterized by progressive increase in pulmonary vascular resistance leading to RV dysfunction. PH is clinically defined by a mPAP of 25 mm Hg or more at rest.[1] Due to diverse processes involved in pathology of pulmonary vasculature, the 5th World Symposium on PH (2013) in Nice, France, recommended classifying PH into five groups[2]:

- PAH
- PH due to left-sided heart disease
- PH due to chronic lung disease and/or chronic hypoxia
- CTEPH
- PH with unclear or multifactorial mechanisms.

The diagnosis of PAH depends upon the detection of elevated PAPs and the exclusion of secondary causes. There exist a variety of methods by which to measure PAP and to assess RV structure and function in the setting of pressure overload. Technical advancements have led to the improvement of these methods, making them easier and more rapid to perform. However, the diagnosis of PH is often made late, with as many as 75% of patients presenting with New York Heart Association (NYHA) Class III or IV and a median time of over 2 years from the onset of symptoms to diagnosis.[3,4] Clinical and echocardiographic parameters such as high NYHA functional class (III or IV), presence of Raynaud's phenomenon, elevated mPAP, elevated mean right atrial pressure, and decreased cardiac index have been associated with worse prognosis.[5] Recent advances in the management of PH, including latest diagnostic and therapeutic options, have led to improved clinical outcomes[6] and studies of early stage PAH demonstrate that earlier intervention with newer pulmonary arterial vasodilating agents provide beneficial effects. Presenting symptoms are nonspecific and often difficult to sort out due to limitations in clinical evaluation. While transthoracic echocardiography has proven to be a useful first step in screening patients suspected of PH, right heart catheterization is required to firmly establish the diagnosis.

A diagnostic approach to the patient with PH is shown in **Figure 3.1**.

Signs and Symptoms

In general, clinical parameters provide limited information as patients usually present with nonspecific symptoms such as exertional dyspnea, fatigue, or weakness. As the disease progresses, patients develop signs and symptoms of progressive heart failure, including peripheral edema, abdominal distension, angina, and lightheadedness or frank syncope. Dyspnea on exertion is the most frequent presenting symptom and is present in >50% of the patients.[1,4] Importantly, chest pain and syncope, which may be considered symptoms that are more consistent with cardiac rather than pulmonary disease states, are each present in approximately 40% of patients.[4] Symptoms typically first occur upon exertion and then subsequently upon rest. Therefore, resting symptoms reflect advanced disease. Symptom severity is assessed using a modified NYHA classification system (**Figure 2.2**). Early stages of PH are often missed, as symptoms are present usually in advanced stage of disease and the mean interval from onset of symptoms to diagnosis of PH is approximately 2 years.[4] Accordingly, the diagnosis of PAH requires a high index of suspicion.

The physical signs of PH depend on the severity of disease. The most common findings in PAH include:
- Left parasternal lift
- Accentuated pulmonary component of second heart sound

- Low frequency pansystolic murmur in lower left sternal border (tricuspid regurgitation)
- High pitched decrescendo murmur occupying the first half of diastole (pulmonary regurgitation)
- Right ventricle third sound.

Jugular venous distension with prominent "a" and "v" wave, peripheral edema, abdominal distension, and hepatomegaly can be seen in advanced stage of disease. Of note, lung auscultation is usually normal.

A meticulous history and a careful physical examination can provide important clues as to the etiology of PH. Signs and symptoms of other systemic disease (eg, scleroderma or other collagen vascular disease, HIV, sarcoidosis, liver disease, congenital heart disease, venous thromboembolism, use of illicit drugs or amphetamine-based diet pills, schistosomiasis, sickle cell disease, etc) should be actively looked for in patients with PH as well as any family history of PH or unexplained cardiac disease. In the presence of clubbing, alternative diagnoses such as congenital heart disease or lung or liver disease should be sought as clubbing is not seen in IPAH.

Diagnostics

■ Electrocardiography

As a screening tool, electrocardiography (EKG) is quite limited as electrocardiographic abnormalities carry a low sensitivity (55%) and low specificity (70%) in patients suspected of PH in general. The most common EKG findings of PH are right ventricular hypertrophy and right axis deviation, which are present in 87% and 79% of patients with PAH, respectively.[4] Findings of right ventricular hypertrophy include:

- Tall R wave in V_1 (R wave/S wave ratio ≥ 1)
- Prominent S waves in leads V_5 and V_6
- Inverted T waves and ST depression in V_1 to V_3
- Right atrial enlargement (prominent P wave in lead II) (**Figure 3.2**).

FIGURE 3.1 — Diagnostic Approach to Pulmonary Hypertension

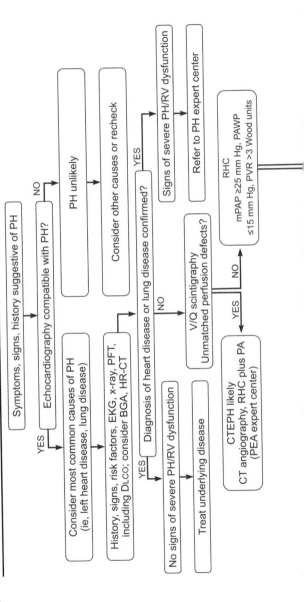

50

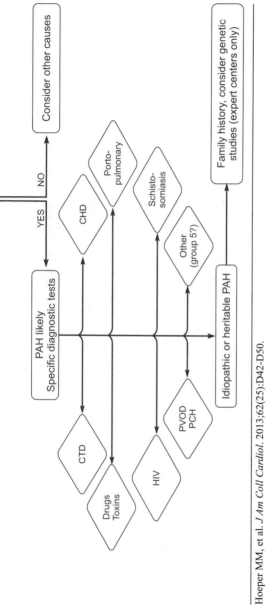

Hoeper MM, et al. *J Am Coll Cardiol.* 2013;62(25):D42-D50.

FIGURE 3.2 — EKG Findings in Patient With Pulmonary Hypertension

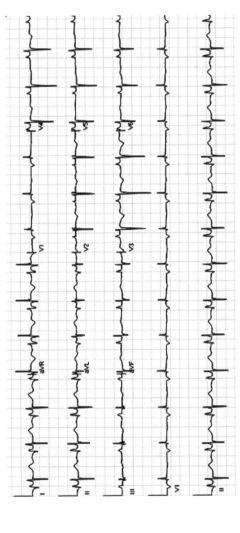

Tall R wave in V_1 (R wave/S wave ratio ≥1), prominent S waves in leads V_5 and V_6, inverted T waves and ST depression in V_1 to V_3, and right atrial enlargement (prominent P wave in lead II).

In late stages of PH, supraventricular arrhythmias including atrial flutter and fibrillation may be present. These findings support the presence of RV hypertrophy and strain and might support the clinical diagnosis of PH in proper clinical setting, but their absences do not exclude presence of PH. Further, EKG changes do not correlate with prognosis and severity of PH.

■ Chest Radiography

Chest radiographs are abnormal in 90% of patients diagnosed with PAH[4] but do not serve as a good screening tool due to poor sensitivity. The classical findings on chest radiograph of a patient with PH include dilated central pulmonary arteries and loss ("pruning") of the peripheral pulmonary vasculature. In advanced cases, diminished retrosternal space and prominent right heart border due to right ventricle and atrial enlargement can be seen. Chest radiograph can also show findings related to underlying lung disease. However, severity of PH does not correlate with the radiographic abnormalities.

■ Echocardiography

Transthoracic echocardiography has become the most useful noninvasive test for evaluating the patient with suspected PH. It is a valuable tool for estimating the PAP, evaluating post-capillary causes of PH, assessing RV size and function, and in monitoring the response to therapy.

In the absence of pulmonic outflow obstruction, pulmonary artery systolic pressure (sPAP) is equal to sum tricuspid regurgitation pressure gradient and right atrial pressure. Tricuspid regurgitation pressure gradient can be calculated by using the modified Bernoulli equation as follows:

$$dP \text{ (mm Hg)} = 4 \times v^2 \text{ (cm}^2)$$

where dP is the tricuspid regurgitation pressure gradient and v is the maximum velocity of the tricuspid valve regurgitant jet, measured by continuous wave Doppler (**Figure 3.3**).

FIGURE 3.3 — Transthoracic Echocardiographic Four-Chamber View

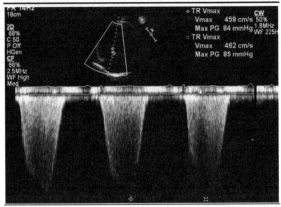

Doppler echocardiography is used to interrogate the tricuspid valve to determine the peak velocity of tricuspid regurgitation jet. The peak tricuspid regurgitation velocity=4.6 m/sec which equates to a peak gradient=85 mm Hg, which when added to an estimation of right atrial pressure will result in estimated pulmonary artery systolic pressure.

The most common technique to estimate the right atrial pressure is based on the diameter and respiratory variation of the inferior vena cava. In case of complete, partial, or no collapse of inferior vena cava with inspiration, right atrial pressure is assumed to be 5, 10, and 15 mm Hg, respectively. Mean PAP can be calculated from sPAP (mean PAP = $0.61 \times$ sPAP+2 mm Hg).

The above method to calculate sPAP is based on the assumption of absence of pulmonic stenosis and presence of an analyzable tricuspid regurgitant jet, which is present in approximately 70% of subjected imaged. Altering the ultrasonographer to the possibility of PH before the study will prompt the ultrasound technician or physician performing the study to spend greater time and attention with regard to interrogating the tricuspid regurgitant jet and evaluating right ventricular function. Use of contrast echocardiography significantly increases the Doppler signal, allowing reliable measurement of peak tricuspid regurgitation velocity in cases where peak tricuspid regurgitation velocity is difficult to measure. Two important caveats are that estimated PAPs are higher in subject with age >50 years and in those with obesity (BMI >30 kg/m^2).[7] In large series of patients, PAP estimated by transthoracic echocardiography correlates well with PAP measured by cardiac catheterization; however, the accuracy of PAP measured by echocardiogram varies considerably. In one study, PAP measured by echocardiogram was within 10 mm Hg of that measured by catheterization only half the time.[8]

Valvular gradients may be underestimated when the Doppler signal is not parallel to the direction of blood flow. Further, in patients with severe tricuspid regurgitation, Doppler-derived sPAP might not be accurate and other echocardiographic parameters that are suggestive of PH independently of tricuspid regurgitation velocity should be considered. Other echocardiographic parameters that suggest presence of PH include RV hypertrophy, paradoxical interventricular septal motion, reduced RV ejection time, increased velocity of pulmonary valve regurgitation, a short acceleration time of right ventricle ejection into the pulmonary artery (PA), reduced collapse of inferior vena cava, and dilated main PA. Significant PH is unusual in the setting of tricuspid regurgitation velocity ≤2.8 m/s and sPAP ≤36 mm Hg, with no additional echocardiographic variables suggestive of PH.[1] On other hand, the presence of tricuspid regurgitation velocity >3.4 m/s, and sPAP <50 mm Hg, with/without additional echocardiographic variables suggestive of PH, make the diagnosis of PH highly likely.[1] As with most diagnostic tests, the sensitivity and negative predictive value of echocardiogram in PH is highly dependent on the risk of PH in the population being studied. In other words, a negative echo in a patient with no known risk factors for PH is reassuring, whereas a patient at increased risk of PH who has unexplained dyspnea may well have PH despite a negative echocardiogram.

The ratio of tricuspid regurgitation velocity (TRV) divided by the velocity-time integral of right ventricular outflow tract (RVOT) as measured by pulsed-wave Doppler tracing (TRV/VTI [RVOT]) has been used to estimate PVR in a noninvasive way.[9] PVR calculated by this approach shows a reasonably good accuracy compared with RHC. However, its use has been questioned in patients with CTEPH.[10]

Assessment of RV function is a critical part of the evaluation of patients with PH and can be done accurately with echocardiography in a noninvasive way (**Figure 3.4**). The myocardial performance index, commonly known as Tei-index, is helpful in assessment of global ventricular function as it incorporates elements

FIGURE 3.4 — Dilation of Right Ventricle

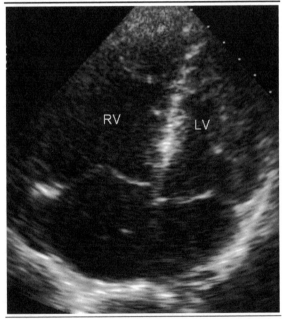

Transthoracic echocardiographic four-chamber view showing marked dilation of the right ventricle in a 47-year-old female with PAH. There is also right atrial dilation.

of both systolic and diastolic phases. Tei-index can be calculated for both left and right ventricles. It is defined as the sum of the isovolumic contraction and the isovolumic relaxation time divided by ejection time. For right ventricle, the normal value of the Tei-index is 0.28 ± 0.04. An increased in right ventricle Tei-index is associated with either PH or left ventricle diastolic abnormalities. Similarly, tricuspid annular plane systolic excursion (TAPSE) is another echocardiographic parameter that estimates RV systolic function. Tei-index and TAPSE are important prognostic parameters in patients with PH.

Echocardiography is also useful in identifying the causes of PH, most common of which is left-sided heart disease. In PH, echocardiography allows reliable assessment of left-sided valvular disease, left ventricular systolic and diastolic dysfunction, and congenital heart disease in a noninvasive way. Therefore, although echocardiography is considered inadequate to establish the diagnosis of PH, it remains a very useful and commonly used screening test.

■ Pulmonary Function Tests

Pulmonary function tests (PFTs) and arterial blood gas are helpful in identifying the underlying lung disease that may be contributing to PH. Decreased forced expiratory volume in one second (FEV_1) and FEV_1 to forced vital capacity (FVC) ratio on PFTs suggest an obstructive disease, whereas low lung volume and normal FEV_1 and FVC indicate presence of restrictive lung disease. Severe obstructive and interstitial lung disease can result in PH; however, in setting of mild obstructive/restrictive pulmonary disease, other explanations for PH should be sought.

The diffusing capacity of the lung for carbon monoxide (DLCO) is usually decreased in patients with PH. Results of arterial blood gas analysis depends of underlying lung disease and typically show mild-to-moderate hypoxemia and mild-to-moderate hypocapnia at rest and during exercise secondary to alveolar hyperventilation.

■ **Ventilation-Perfusion Scan**

Ventilation-perfusion (V/Q) scanning should be performed in essentially all patients with PAH to exclude the possibility of chronic thromboembolic disease, as CTEPH is treated differently than PAH and is potentially reversible with surgery. Furthermore, up to half of patients with CTEPH have no history of venous thromboembolism and are unable to recall symptoms suggestive of acute pulmonary embolism. V/Q scanning has a higher sensitivity for excluding CTEPH than CT pulmonary angiogram, and a normal or low probability V/Q scan makes the diagnosis of chronic thromboembolic disease unlikely. If CTEPH is detected by V/Q scan, pulmonary angiography and CT angiography (*see below*) is helpful to define the extent and type of thromboembolic pulmonary disease. The V/Q scan may also reveal the presence of intra-cardiac or pulmonary to systemic shunts. Patients with known PH or right to left shunts should be discussed with the radiologist prior to study to allow modification, if necessary, of the amount of aggregated albumin used.

■ **Computerized Tomography**

High-resolution computerized tomography (CT) scanning of chest is a useful, noninvasive test for evaluation of lung parenchyma and to identify underlying lung pathology (**Table 3.1**). Centrilobular ground-glass nodules are commonly seen in patients with IPAH. Neovascularity can be seen in severe cases of PH. Features such as interstitial edema, thickening of interlobular septa, pleural effusion, and lymphadenopathy suggest the presence of pulmonary veno-occlusive disease.

Contrast CT angiography of the PA is useful in delineating the anatomic detail of the pulmonary vasculature and evaluation of CTEPH. PA dilation is a hallmark finding of increased PAP. The presence of bronchial arterial collaterals, partial or complete luminal obstruction, intraluminal abnormalities of the pulmonary vessels, and mosaic attenuation of the pulmonary parenchyma can be seen in CTEPH. Although

TABLE 3.1 — Causes of Pulmonary Hypertension and Associated Imaging Findings

Shunt (ASD, VSD, PDA)	Direct visualization of shunt
	Shunt vascularity (overcirculation)
Pulmonary fibrosis	Reticular opacities (inter- and intralobular septal thickening, honeycomb cysts)
	Traction bronchiectasis
COPD	Emphysema
HIV	Opportunistic infection
Hepatopulmonary syndrome	Linear opacities extending to pleura
Mediastinal fibrosis	Infiltration of mediastinal fat
	Calcified and noncalcified lymph nodes
	Narrowing of mediastinal structures
PVOD	Pulmonary edeoma
	Pleural effusions
	Mediastinal lymphadenopathy
Capillary hemangiomatosis	Centrilobular ground glass nodules
	Hemorrhagic pleural effusion

contrast CT angiography is a reliable and accurate test to delineate central pulmonary vasculature, it has low sensitivity to evaluate segmental level and smaller vasculature.

Traditional pulmonary angiography is still performed before pulmonary endarterectomy to delineate the pulmonary vasculature. In experienced centers, pulmonary angiography can be performed without any major adverse hemodynamic effects using modern contrast media and selective injections. Typical angiographic findings in CTEPH include abrupt narrowing of the major pulmonary arteries, obstruction of vessels near their origin with absence of blood flow to respective lung segments, pouch defects, webs or bands, and intimal irregularities.

■ Cardiac Magnetic Resonance

Cardiac magnetic resonance (CMR) is considered as the gold standard in the morphologic and functional evaluation of the heart. It has become the first-line imaging modality for the assessment of many types of congenital and acquired cardiovascular disorders.

The use of CMR in diagnosis and management of PH and RV failure remains an area of active investigation. Diagnostic accuracy of CMR to assess the RV size, morphology, and function, and hemodynamic changes has been validated in several studies.[11,12] Hemodynamic data obtained from CMR, especially increased RV end-diastolic volume, can be used as a marker for progressive RV failure in the follow-up. Patients with PH have higher RV mass, which is due to an increase mPAP and PVR leading to remodeling and compensatory RV hypertrophy. Although CMR is potentially helpful in clinical decision-making and follow-up of patients with PH, its role in managing PAH has yet to be determined.

Evaluation of the RV Function by CMR

Ventricular epicardial and endocardial borders are outlined on each end-diastolic short axis slice image. Myocardial volume is then calculated by multiplying the area between these outlines by the slice thickness. The product of the density of myocardium and the sum total of the myocardial slice volumes for each ventricle thus give an estimate of left end-diastolic ventricular mass and right end-diastolic ventricular mass. Ventricular mass index (VMI) is calculated by dividing right end-diastolic ventricular mass by the left end-diastolic ventricular mass. It is one of the most commonly used CMR parameters to assess the RV functional changes and correlates well with parameters derived from RHC.

Although CMR has emerged as a potential tool to improve the diagnostic accuracy for PH, for evaluation of mild PH, CMR should be combined with other imaging modalities as it tends to underestimate the PH, especially if PH is not associated with any structural heart disease. While CMR is expensive, its noninvasive nature allows for serial testing during longitudinal follow-up. However, cost-effectiveness of CMR in evaluating and managing PH need further investigation.

■ Biomarkers

Routine biochemistry, including liver function test, hematology, and thyroid function tests, are required in all patients with PH. American (ACC/AHA) and European guidelines recommend serological testing for connective tissue disease and testing for hepatitis and HIV in cases of unexplained PAH. Recently, the potential role of various other biomarkers in diagnosis and prognosis of PAH has described. These include markers of heart failure, endothelial dysfunction, platelet dysfunction, cardiac myocyte damage, and oxidative stress.

The most commonly used biomarker for diagnosing and monitoring PAH is brain natriuretic peptide (BNP). BNP is derived from proBNP after its breakdown into biologically inactive N-terminal segment (NT-proBNP) and BNP. Elevated serum NT-proBNP and BNP levels are nonspecific markers for left and right ventricular stress and, in isolation, are not diagnostic of a specific disease. While elevated BNP is often used to support the diagnosis of left-sided congestive heart failure in patients presenting with dyspnea, NT-proBNP and BNP levels are increased in patients with renal insufficiency and anemia and are lower in patients with obesity. Thus, BNP has limited utility in screening preclinical PAH in asymptomatic patients with low pretest probability. However, for patients suspected of having PAH with elevated sPAP by echo, additional testing with the biomarker BNP (or NT proBNP) might provide incremental value in identifying patients who do not have PAH compared with echo sPAP alone.

In patients with known baseline NT-proBNP and/or BNP, an elevation in levels may indicate acute RV decompensation and can be used to monitoring RV failure due to PH. BNP levels can be used to assess severity of PH as it correlates with exercise capacity, NYHA functional class, and various hemodynamic parameters of PH. BNP has also been evaluated to assess prognosis in PAH with higher levels indicating worse clinical outcomes.[13] NT-proBNP is more stable with a longer half-life, hence it is better suited to measure in lab. Recent studies have shown decrease in levels of NT-proBNP with treatment; however, cut-off levels for NT-proBNP to be used in clinical practice are still under investigation.

■ Right Heart Catheterization and Vasodilatory Testing

While transthoracic echocardiography is an important screening tool for assessing PH, RHC is the gold standard for diagnosis of PH and is mandatory whenever PH is suspected. PAH refers to a subgroup of PH, defined hemodynamically as mPAP ≥25 mm Hg, PAWP ≤15 mm Hg, and PVR >3 Wood units.

A small percentage of PAH patients have disease that is characterized more by increased pulmonary vascular tone than an obliterative pulmonary vasculopathy. The majority of these patients respond extremely well to calcium-channel blockers (CCBs) and have a significantly better prognosis. To identify which patients are likely to respond to CCB therapy, acute pulmonary vasodilator testing should be performed in patients with IPAH.[14] Intravenous adenosine, intravenous epoprostenol, or inhaled NO are the standard agents used for vasoreactivity testing in patients with IPAH. A near normalization of pulmonary hemodynamics is needed before patients can be considered for therapy with

CCBs. By convention, a near normalization of pulmonary hemodynamics has been defined as a decrease in mPAP of 10 mm Hg or greater to a mPAP <40 mm Hg with no decrease in cardiac output.

RHC with vasodilator testing should be performed in hemodynamically stable patients at centers experienced in vasoreactivity testing. The risks of vasodilator testing are similar to the risks of RHC and have a low morbidity and mortality of 1.1% and 0.055%, respectively.[15] The European guidelines recommend that testing should be done at the time of RHC in a referral testing center.[1]

Less than 10% of PAH patients have a long-term response to CCB therapy, and most of the data supporting vasodilator testing recommendations comes from studies on patients with PAH.[16,17] American (ACC/AHA) and European guidelines do not recommend vasodilator testing in other groups of PH (Groups 2, 3, 4, and 5).[1,16] Using inhaled nitric oxide (iNO) and intravenous epoprostenol as agents for vasodilator testing, it was shown that in drug-induced PAH, HIV-associated PAH, and PAH with porto-pulmonary hypertension, an acute response predicted a sustained response to CCBs. However, in PAH due to connective tissue disease, pulmonary veno-occlusive disease (PVOD), pulmonary capillary hemangiomatosis (PCH), and congenital heart disease, an acute response is not predictive of long-term response and initiation of CCB therapy may lead to clinical deterioration.[18]

The following are indications for vasodilator testing:

- In IPAH or acquired PAH to evaluate treatment options
- Complicated congenital heart disease with severe PAH to determine the next best step in management
- Prior to Fontan (atriopulmonary connection) surgery or one of its modifications, with elevated PVR
- In heart transplantation candidates to assess the need for concomitant lung transplantation.

Baseline measurements of the hemodynamic variables including central venous pressure, right atrial pressure, systolic and diastolic right ventricular pressure, systolic and diastolic PAP, mPAP, PVR, PVR index, PCWP, cardiac output (measured by thermodilution or by the Fick method), cardiac index, stroke volume, systolic and diastolic systemic blood pressure, mean arterial pressure, systemic resistance, systemic resistance index, systemic oxygen saturation, and mixed venous oxygen saturation are obtained to determine initial values. These variables are then measured again after infusion of a vasodilator agent. In some patients, hemodynamic variables are repeated after exercise or intravascular expansion to look for exercise-induced PH or left ventricular diastolic dysfunction.

Initial baseline hemodynamic values are compared with the values obtained after infusion of vasodilator agent. A positive vasodilator test is defined as a decrease in PAP of at least 10 mm Hg, a pulmonary artery systolic pressure of <40 mm Hg, and a preserved or increased cardiac output.[1,16] This new definition led to an increased specificity compared with the previous definition, where a positive test was defined by reduction in both mean PAP and PVR by >20% with use of vasodilator.[19]

Conclusion

PH has been defined by an elevated PAP. With the development of new therapies for PH screening, prompt diagnosis and accurate assessment of PH severity have become increasingly important. In patients with clinically suspected PH EKG, chest radiograph, transthoracic echocardiogram, pulmonary function tests, and high-resolution chest CT can provide important initial diagnostic information and be helpful in directing further diagnostic workup (**Figure 3.5**).

**FIGURE 3.5 — Short Axis View of
Left and Right Ventricles**

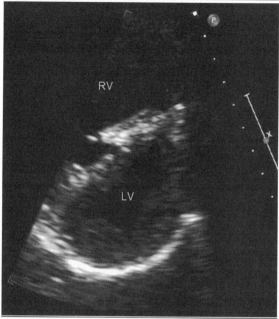

Transthoracic echocardiography short axis view of the left
and right ventricles. The right ventricle is dilated causing
leftward displacement of the interventricular septum. This
confers a "D" rather than a "donut" shape of the left ventricle.

Key Points

- Early diagnosis of PH requires a high level of
  suspicion, and practitioners should consider
  the diagnosis in any patient with dyspnea on
  exertion that is not readily explained by another
  disease or condition.
- Transthoracic echocardiography is a useful
  screening tool in patients with suspected PH, but
  cannot exclude the diagnosis and should not be
  considered as evidence of a definitive diagnosis.

- Other diagnostic tests that are useful in determining the risk and etiology of PH include:
  - PFTs
  - V/Q scan
  - Serology
  - Biomarkers such as BNP/NT-proBNP
  - Sleep study
  - High-resolution chest CT or pulmonary angiography
  - CMR
- Right heart catheterization (RHC) is necessary to confirm the diagnosis of PAH and determine the severity of right ventricular compromise.
- To identify patients who will respond to vasodilators, acute vasodilator testing should be performed during RHC in patients with IPAH.

REFERENCES

1. Bogaard HJ, Condliffe R, Frantz R, et al. Definitions and diagnosis of pulmonary hypertension. *J Am Coll Cardiol.* 2013;62(25 suppl):D42-D50.

2. Simonneau G, Gatzoulis MA, Adatia I, et al. Updated clinical classification of pulmonary hypertension. *J Am Coll Cardiol.* 2013;62(25 suppl):D34-D41.

3. Humbert M, Sitbon O, Chaouat A, et al. Survival in patients with idiopathic, familial, and anorexigen-associated pulmonary arterial hypertension in the modern management era. *Circulation.* 2010;122(2):156-163.

4. Rich S, Dantzker DR, Ayres SM, et al. Primary pulmonary hypertension. A national prospective study. *Ann Intern Med.* 1987;107(2):216-223.

5. D'Alonzo GE, Barst RJ, Ayres SM, et al. Survival in patients with primary pulmonary hypertension. Results from a national prospective registry. *Ann Intern Med.* 1991;115(5):343-349.

6. Galiè N, Manes A, Negro L, Palazzini M, Bacchi-Reggiani ML, Branzi A. A meta-analysis of randomized controlled trials in pulmonary arterial hypertension. *Eur Heart J.* 2009;30:394-403.

7. D'Andrea A, Naeije R, Grünig E, et al. Echocardiography of the pulmonary circulation and right ventricular function: exploring the physiologic spectrum in 1,480 normal subjects. *Chest.* 2014;145(5):1071-1078.

8. Fisher MR, Forfia PR, Chamera E, et al. Accuracy of Doppler echocardiography in the hemodynamic assessment of pulmonary hypertension. *Am J Respir Crit Care Med.* 2009; 179(7):615-621.

9. Farzaneh-Far R, Na B, Whooley MA, et al. Usefulness of non-invasive estimate of pulmonary vascular resistance to predict mortality, heart failure, and adverse cardiovascular events in patients with stable coronary artery disease (from the Heart and Soul Study). *Am J Cardiol.* 2008;101(6):762-766.

10. Xie Y, Burke BM, Kopelnik A, et al. Echocardiographic estimation of pulmonary vascular resistance in chronic thromboembolic pulmonary hypertension: utility of right heart Doppler measurements. *Echocardiography.* 2014;31(1):29-33.

11. Wang N, Hu X, Liu C, et al. A systematic review of the diagnostic accuracy of cardiovascular magnetic resonance for pulmonary hypertension. *Can J Cardiol.* 2014;30(4):455-463.

3

12. Ibrahim el-SH, White RD. Cardiovascular magnetic resonance for the assessment of pulmonary arterial hypertension: toward a comprehensive CMR exam. *Magn Reson Imaging.* 2012;30(8):1047-1058.

13. Fijalkowska A, Kurzyna M, Torbicki A, et al. Serum N-terminal brain natriuretic peptide as a prognostic parameter in patients with pulmonary hypertension. *Chest.* 2006;129:1313-1321.

14. Morales-Blanhir J, Santos S, de Jover L, et al. Clinical value of vasodilator test with inhaled nitric oxide for predicting long-term response to oral vasodilators in pulmonary hypertension. *Respiratory Medicine.* 2004;98(3):225-234.

15. Hoeper MM, Lee SH, Voswinckel R, et al. Complications of right heart catheterization procedures in patients with pulmonary hypertension in experienced centers. *J Am Coll Cardiol.* 2006;48(12):2546-2552.

16. McLaughlin VV, Archer SL, Badesch DB, et al. ACCF/AHA 2009 expert consensus document on pulmonary hypertension a report of the American College of Cardiology Foundation Task Force on Expert Consensus Documents and the American Heart Association developed in collaboration with the American College of Chest Physicians; American Thoracic Society, Inc.; and the Pulmonary Hypertension Association. *J Am Coll Cardiol.* 2009;53(17):1573-1619.

17. Sitbon O, Humbert M, Jaïs X, et al. Long-term response to calcium channel blockers in idiopathic pulmonary arterial hypertension. *Circulation.* 2005;111(23):3105-3111.

18. Montani D, Savale L, Natali D, et al. Long-term response to calcium-channel blockers in non-idiopathic pulmonary arterial hypertension. *Eur Heart J.* 2010;31(15):1898-1907.

19. Tonelli AR, Alnuaimat H, Mubarak K. Pulmonary vasodilator testing and use of calcium channel blockers in pulmonary arterial hypertension. *Respir Med.* 2010;104(4):481-496.

4

Radiologic Approaches

by Daniel Green, MD and
Rakesh Shah, MD

Right heart catheterization (RHC) is the diagnostic gold standard for PAH, but its invasive approach and expense prohibit its routine use for screening populations at risk. Transthoracic echocardiography with Doppler ultrasound is a noninvasive way to estimate PAP and has become the most frequently used modality for diagnosing PH.

While chest radiography and CT do not directly evaluate PAP, they provide anatomic information about the heart and main pulmonary artery. Identification of morphologic changes secondary to increased PVR suggests the diagnosis of PH with high accuracy.[1-4] In addition, by providing excellent detail of smaller pulmonary artery branches and the lung parenchyma, CT is particularly useful in clarifying an underlying cause when present. Although the widespread nature of these examinations can incidentally detect early signs of PH in patients undergoing testing for other reasons, their sensitivity for excluding PAH is low and a lack of findings suggestive of PH does not exclude the diagnosis.

The characteristic morphologic findings of PH are dilatation of the central pulmonary arteries and abrupt tapering of more peripheral branches. Signs of PH in advanced cases include right atrial and ventricular dilatation, right ventricular hypertrophy, and leftward shift of the interventricular septum. Pericardial effusion occurs in severe cases and portends a poor prognosis.[5] These general features are present in PH of any cause. Specific findings for particular diagnoses will be addressed later.

On chest radiography, main pulmonary artery size is best evaluated on a frontal view. In between the left heart border and aortic knob, the normal lung-mediastinum interface is concave. An enlarged main pulmonary artery alters this contour forming a convexity (**Figure 4.1**). Measurement of the descending right pulmonary artery has been described but is difficult and unreliable.[2] Increased lucency of the lung fields may represent peripheral oligemia secondary to diminished vascularity. Asymmetric lucency has been described in pulmonary embolism (the Westermark sign). Right atrial enlargement is apparent on a frontal view as lateral displacement of the right heart border, and an enlarged right ventricle fills the retrosternal space on a lateral view.

FIGURE 4.1 — Pulmonary Hypertension

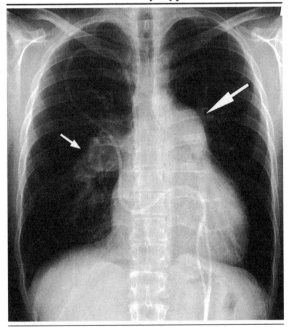

Chest radiograph shows enlargement of the main pulmonary artery *(large arrow)* as well as the right *(small arrow)* and left pulmonary arteries.

The two most widely accepted measures for predicting elevated PAP on non–EKG-gated chest CT are the transverse diameter of the main pulmonary artery (dPA) and the ratio of the transverse diameters of the main pulmonary artery and ascending aorta at the level of the bifurcation of the right pulmonary artery (rPA). Both are easily measured on an axial CT slice and reproducible with or without intravenous contrast. Measurement of the ascending aorta serves as a control for the effect of body surface area and the cardiac cycle on pulmonary artery size.

Patients with dPA >29 mm have a higher likelihood of dyspnea than those with dPA <29 mm.[6] By combining cutoffs of dPA >29 mm and rPA >1, CT has a high positive predictive value for PH. In one study, a segmental pulmonary artery to bronchus ratio >1 in three or four lobes increased specificity to 100%.[1] The rPA is the most accurate of these measures in patients younger than 50 years, but the accuracy decreases in older patients because aortic size tends to increase with age. It is also important to keep in mind that dPA <29 mm and rPA <1 each have a low negative predictive value and do not imply the absence of PH.[2]

CT angiography is excellent at showing other findings of PH, such as abruptly tapered peripheral pulmonary artery branches with a beaded appearance and tortuous course (**Figure 4.2**). Right ventricular hypertrophy is apparent when myocardial thickness reaches 4 to 5 mm (**Figure 4.2**). Right ventricular enlargement is characterized by bowing of the interventricular septum toward the left ventricle and right ventricular chamber size exceeding that of the left ventricle.

Similar measurements and observations can be made on MRI. Volumetric analysis of the right heart and pulmonary arteries using more advanced EKG-gated CT and MRI functions will not be discussed in this chapter.

FIGURE 4.2 — Idiopathic Pulmonary Hypertension

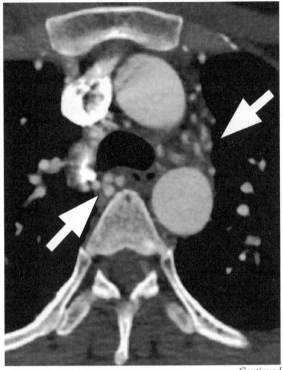

Continued

Idiopathic Pulmonary Hypertension

Beyond the essential CT and radiographic findings of PH, additional imaging features of idiopathic PH can be separated into vascular and parenchymal categories[3] (**Table 4.1**).

Small tortuous peripheral vessels corresponding to the histopathologic finding of plexogenic arteriopathy are the hallmark of IPAH (**Figure 4.2**). Eccentric intraluminal thrombi are not typical but may be seen in severe cases due to high pressure and turbulent flow.

FIGURE 4.2 — *Continued*

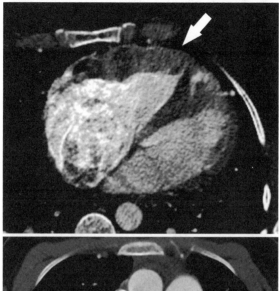

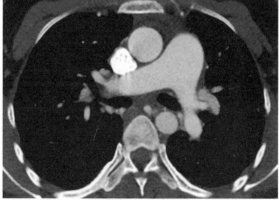

Enlarged main pulmonary artery, collateral vessels in the mediastinum *(large arrows)*, and severe hypertrophy of right ventricular myocardium *(small arrow)*.

Calcification of the pulmonary arteries may also occur in severe cases.

Mosaic attenuation of the lungs, signifying regional variations in perfusion with sharply demarcated areas of normal and low attenuation parenchyma, is the main parenchymal finding in idiopathic disease

TABLE 4.1 — General Imaging Features of Pulmonary Hypertension

Radiography
- Enlarged main pulmonary artery (PA)
- Increased lucency of lungs
- Right atrial and ventricular enlargement

CT
- Enlarged main pulmonary artery
- Increased main PA to ascending aorta ratio
- Increased segmental PA to bronchus ratio
- Tapered peripheral pulmonary artery branches
- Right ventricular hypertrophy
- Right atrial and ventricular enlargement
- Inversion of the interventricular septum

(**Figure 4.3**). Low attenuation regions correspond to hypoperfused lung secondary either to occluded arteries or vasculopathy of nonoccluded arteries.[7] Areas of normal attenuation may be supplied by vessels of increased caliber.

Mosaic attenuation is present in PH of several different causes, particularly CTEPH and pulmonary veno-occlusive disease (PVOD). Minimum-intensity projections increase the sensitivity of detection.[8] The absence of air trapping on expiratory CT can help to differentiate vascular etiologies of mosaic attenuation from airway diseases.

Chronic Thromboembolic Disease

Like idiopathic PH, CTEPH has both vascular and parenchymal findings. In addition to the typical pulmonary artery and right heart alterations, the most specific vascular findings for chronic thromboembolic disease are partial filling defects of the pulmonary arteries on CT angiography (**Figure 4.4** and **Table 4.2**). The result of incomplete resolution of acute pulmonary emboli, organized intraluminal thrombi have several appearances. Recanalized clot eccentrically lines the arterial wall and becomes endothelialized, resulting in abrupt

FIGURE 4.3 — Mosaic Attenuation

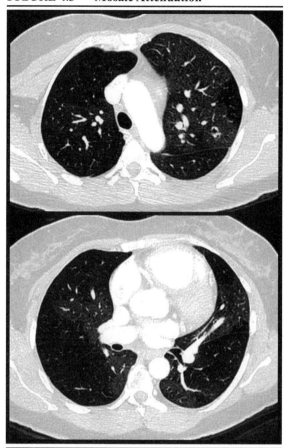

Axial CT images demonstrate patchy areas of lucency and ground glass attenuation.

luminal narrowing and occasionally calcification. Bands are linear filling defects, and webs are networks of linear filling defects, usually in lobar or segmental branches rather than the higher caliber main pulmonary arteries[9] (**Figure 4.5**). Some experts favor ventilation perfusion scanning as part of the workup for CTEPH (see *Chapter 11*).

FIGURE 4.4 — Chronic Thromboembolic Disease

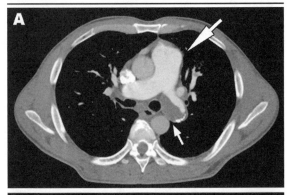

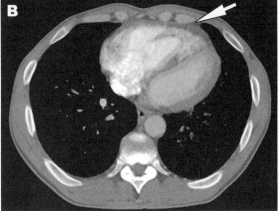

Figure A shows enlarged main pulmonary artery *(large arrow)* and partially calcified eccentric filling defect in left pulmonary artery *(small arrow)*. **Figure B** shows mild right ventricular hypertrophy *(arrow)* and absence of left lower lobe pulmonary arteries.

Attenuation of pulmonary arteries occurs in the distribution distal to unresolved thromboemboli, which is typically asymmetric. This is in contrast to the more symmetric pruning of the pulmonary arterial tree that occurs in other forms of PH.

The development of collateral systemic-to-pulmonary arterial shunting—typically via the bronchial,

TABLE 4.2 — Causes of Pulmonary Hypertension and Associated Findings: IPH vs CTEPH

	IPH	CTEPH
Vascular	• Symmetric pruning of pulmonary arteries • Collateral less frequent	• Segmental pruning of pulmonary arteries • Collateral more frequent • Partial filling defects (eg, eccentric clot, bands, webs)
Parenchymal	• Nonsegmental mosaic attenuation	• Segmental mosaic attenuation • Peripheral scarring

intercostal, internal mammary, and abdominal arteries—more frequently occurs in chronic thromboembolic disease than idiopathic PH (73% compared with 14%) but can be seen in both entities.[10]

Parenchymal findings include mosaic attenuation of the lungs and peripheral scarring from prior pulmonary infarcts (**Figure 4.6**). Mosaic attenuation occurs more often in chronic thromboembolic disease than in idiopathic PH.[11] Unlike nonembolic forms of PH, the distribution of mosaic attenuation in embolic disease tends to be segmental with lucent areas of lung occurring in areas affecting by chronic emboli.[8] Scarring can be wedge-shaped, linear, nodular, or cavitary. Despite its variable appearance, it is always peripherally situated and may be associated with pleural thickening.[10]

Tumor thromboemboli and intravenous talcosis cause similar findings as chronic thromboembolic disease but are exceedingly rare.

Congenital Shunt

Eisenmenger syndrome is an irreversible form of PAH that develops as a result of longstanding systemic-to-pulmonary shunting (**Table 4.3**). The most common congenital causes are atrial septal defect, ventricular septal defect, patent ductus arteriosus, and

FIGURE 4.5 — Pulmonary Webs

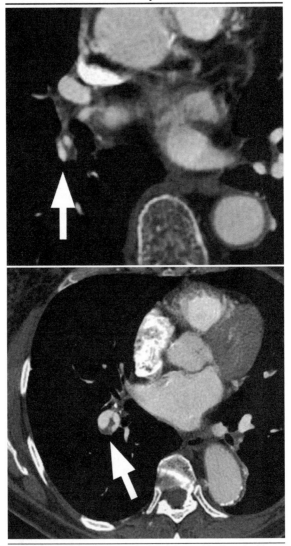

Examples of pulmonary webs in patient with chronic thromboembolic disease.

FIGURE 4.6 — Chronic Thromboembolic Disease

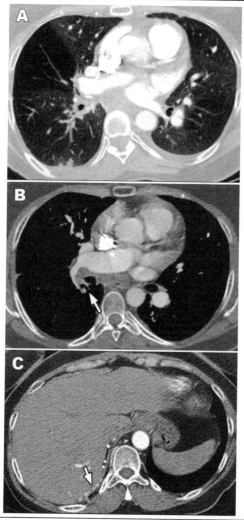

Segmental mosaic attenuation *(A)*, eccentric clot in the right pulmonary artery *(B)*, and collateral vessels in the lower right hemithorax *(C)*.

TABLE 4.3 — Other Causes of Pulmonary Hypertension and Associated Findings

Cause	Findings
Eisenmenger syndrome shunts (ASK, VSD, PDA)	Direct visualization of shunt
	Shunt vascularity or overcirculation
Pulmonary fibrosis	Reticular opacities consisting of inter- and intralobular septal thickening, honeycomb cysts, and traction bronchiectasis
COPD	Emphysema
HIV	Opportunistic infection
Hepatopulmonary syndrome	Cirrhosis
	Linear opacities extending to pleura
Mediastinal fibrosis	Calcified and noncalcified nodes
	Infiltration of mediastinal fat
	Narrowing of mediastinal structures
PVOD	Pulmonary edema, pleural effusion, and mediastinal lymphadenopathy
Capillary hemangiomatosis	Centrilobular ground glass nodule and hemorrhagic pleural effusion

partial anomalous pulmonary venous return (**Figure 4.7**). Pulmonary vascular remodeling and elevated PAP occurs in response to the increase in blood flow through the pulmonary circulation. If left uncorrected, approximately 50% of patients with a large VSD (>1 cm) and 10% of patients with a large ASD (>2 cm) will eventually develop PH.[12] Sinus venosus ASD, which is associated with PAPVR, is associated with a higher risk than primum or secundum ASD.

Indirect signs on chest radiography include an enlarged main pulmonary artery and prominent linear opacities emanating from the hila corresponding to enlarged pulmonary artery branches, collectively referred to as shunt vascularity.

Along with the stereotypic changes of PH, the characteristic CT finding of shunt vascularity is an increase in the size and number of the pulmonary artery and its branches, the result of pulmonary overcirculation. Dilated central pulmonary arteries may develop atherosclerotic disease and calcification. Intravenous contrast may directly identify the shunt. Mosaic attenuation of the lungs is present in a small percentage of cases.[8]

Phase contrast MRI can quantify systemic-to-pulmonary arterial shunting by measuring the ratio of flow through the pulmonary arteries (Qp) to flow through the aorta (Qs). In the absence of shunting, Qp:Qs ratio is equal to 1. A Qp:Qs >1.5 is more likely to cause pulmonary hypertension, and a Qp:Qs >2 is more likely to result in Eisenmenger syndrome.[13,14] A Qp:Qs <1.5 is unlikely to be hemodynamically significant.[14]

Pulmonary arteriovenous malformations (PAVMs) are another type of shunt that has been associated with PAH. For the degree of shunting to be severe enough to be hemodynamically significant, several vascular malformations must be present, which is highly suggestive of hereditary hemorrhagic telangiectasias (HHT) also known as Osler-Weber-Rendu syndrome. Contrast-enhanced CT demonstrates the anomalous communication of pulmonary arteries to veins without an intervening capillary bed, as well as in other organs such as the liver. HHT is caused by mutations in the gene for endoglin or activin receptor-like kinase-1 (ACVRL1). The cause of PAH in this syndrome is unclear. PAH is strongly associated with mutations in the gene for bone morphogenic protein receptor-2 (BMPR-2) which is not associated with PAVMs, is in the same superfamily of transforming growth factor beta receptors as endoglin and ACVRL1, suggesting that PAH in HHT may be caused by abnormalities of

**FIGURE 4.7 — Congenital Shunts in
Two Different Patients**

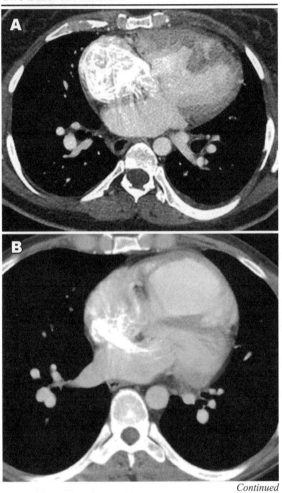

Continued

FIGURE 4.7 — *Continued*

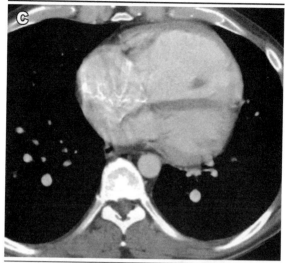

Ventricular septal defect and severe right ventricular hypertrophy *(A)*. Injected contrast flows from the right to the left atrium through an atrial septal defect *(B)* and right ventricular enlargement *(C)*. These findings suggest Eisenmenger physiology.

pulmonary vascular remodeling rather than increased pulmonary blood flow.

Pulmonary Fibrosis

Pulmonary fibrosis of any etiology is characterized on CT by symmetrically decreased lung volumes, interlobular septal thickening, and traction bronchiectasis (**Figure 4.8**). Distribution of these findings and other additional findings vary with the underlying cause.

Idiopathic fibrosis is characterized by the usual interstitial pneumonia (UIP) pattern—peripheral and basilar predominance with progression of subpleural honeycombing (**Figure 4.9**). The fibrotic variant of nonspecific idiopathic pneumonia (NSIP) also has a peripheral and basilar distribution; however, honey-

FIGURE 4.8 — Pulmonary Fibrosis

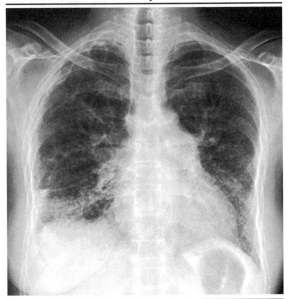

Chest radiograph shows enlarged main pulmonary artery and bibasilar reticular opacities.

Continued

combing is rare and ground glass opacities are more likely to develop. When present, subpleural sparing is highly suggestive of NSIP.

Collagen vascular diseases are the most common cause of pulmonary fibrosis–related PH, typically presenting with an NSIP-like pattern, although a UIP-like pattern can predominate. PH arises independently of the presence of pulmonary parenchymal disease. Scleroderma, the most likely of the collagen vascular diseases to affect PAP,[15] may present with ancillary findings of a dilated esophagus and soft tissue calcifications.

Sarcoidosis can also cause pulmonary fibrosis; although like the collagen vascular diseases, PH can develop without parenchymal disease. Pulmonary fibrosis secondary to sarcoidosis includes both stage 3

FIGURE 4.8 — *Continued*

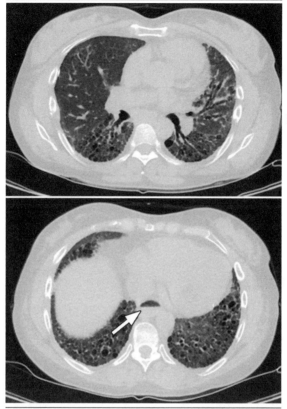

4

CT images confirm the findings and show dilatation of the esophagus *(arrow)* suggestive of scleroderma.

and stage 4 disease. Findings at radiography and CT are centrally distributed, preferentially affecting the upper lungs (**Figure 4.10**). Centrilobular and perilymphatic calcified and noncalcified lung nodules represent noncaseating granulomas. Calcified or non-calcified mediastinal and hilar lymphadenopathy is common.

In patients with pulmonary fibrosis, the development of PH is a poor prognostic indicator[16]; however, there is no correlation with CT-determined severity of

FIGURE 4.9 — Idiopathic Pulmonary Fibrosis

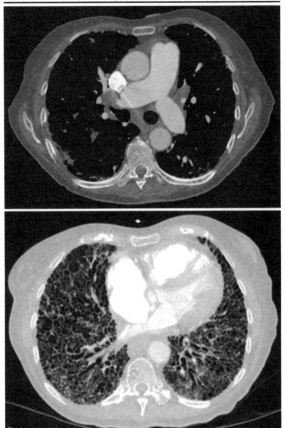

Continued

pulmonary fibrosis. Unlike other causes of PH, there is no consistent correlation with main pulmonary artery diameter.[1,17,18] Even in the absence of PH, the main pulmonary artery enlarges in the setting of fibrosis, possibly through a traction effect.[17,18] In these patients, rPA is a more accurate indicator.[16]

FIGURE 4.9 — *Continued*

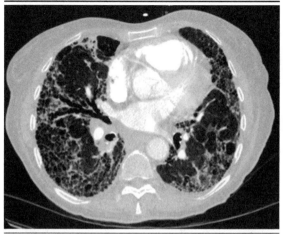

Dilatation of the main pulmonary artery and extensive inter-lobular septal thickening and traction bronchiectasis.

Chronic Obstructive Pulmonary Disease

When CT demonstrates an enlarged main pulmo-nary artery in the setting of emphysema, the positive predictive value for PH is high.[1,19] Like pulmonary fibrosis, the extent of parenchymal emphysema does not correlate with the severity of PH.

Pulmonary Langerhans Cell Histiocytosis

Pulmonary Langerhans cell histiocytosis (PLCH) is a smoking-related lung disease that commonly results in PH.[20] Although it is a multi-organ disease, involvement is usually limited to the lungs. The typical CT findings are peribronchiolar nodules and air cysts that predominate in the upper portions of the lungs.[21] When centrilobular ground glass nodules are present, they likely correspond to respiratory bronchiolitis (RB)

FIGURE 4.10 — Sarcoidosis

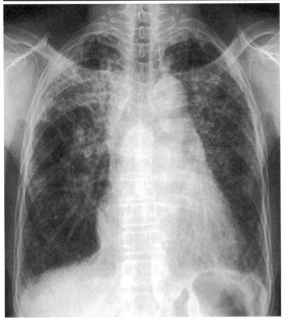

Continued

or respiratory bronchiolitis interstitial lung disease (RB-ILD).[21] As the disease progresses, nodules cavitate and become cystic. The presence of cysts with well-defined walls helps differentiate from the lucent areas of emphysema, which have imperceptible walls. The cystic spaces of PLCH can also be mistaken for another cystic lung disease—lymphangioleiomyomatosis (LAM). Cysts in PLCH tend to be irregularly shaped and spare the lung bases, while cysts in LAM are round and do not spare the bases. LAM can also result in PH, although less frequently than PLCH does.

HIV

PAH occurs in approximately 0.5% of patients with HIV infection. An enlarged main pulmonary artery

FIGURE 4.10 — *Continued*

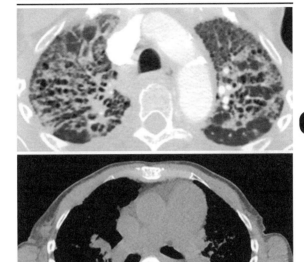

4

Chest radiograph and CT show symmetric reticular opacities in both upper lobes as well as dilatation of the main pulmonary artery.

with evidence of opportunistic infection, lymphoma, or Kaposi's sarcoma is suggestive of the diagnosis.

Hepatopulmonary Syndrome

Approximately 2% to 3% of patients with cirrhosis develop portopulmonary hypertension. Most patients have evidence of cirrhosis on imaging, and many have signs of portal hypertension, such as varices and splenomegaly. The main pulmonary artery is not necessarily enlarged.[22]

The other characteristic imaging findings are dilated terminal pulmonary artery branches that extend to the pleura rather than tapering, corresponding to intrapulmonary arteriovenous shunting. These findings manifest as bilateral reticulonodular opacities at the lung bases on radiography, often mimicking pulmonary fibrosis. On CT, they represent dilated distal arteries that can be differentiated from septal lines by their centrilobular location. The absence of honeycombing and traction bronchiectasis also helps to distinguish this entity from pulmonary fibrosis.

Mediastinal Fibrosis

Two types of mediastinal fibrosis have been described: localized (82%) and diffuse (18%).[23] Each has a distinct CT appearance, although both are characterized by dense proliferation of fibrotic tissue replacing the mediastinal fat and surrounding mediastinal structures (**Figure 4.11**). PH results from extrinsic compression of the central pulmonary arteries or veins.

Localized mediastinal disease is more likely to develop scattered calcifications and tends to affect the right paratracheal and subcarinal regions. Etiology is believed to be the late sequelae of an abnormal immune response to the fungus *Histoplasma capsulatum*, but tuberculosis or other fungal infections may also serve as culprits.[24] The diffuse form is a more infiltrative and ill-defined soft tissue mass replacing the mediastinal fat without calcification.[23] It is thought to be associated with autoimmune disorders or other idiopathic fibroinflammatory disorders, such as retroperitoneal fibrosis.[24]

Intravenous contrast is helpful in delineating the mediastinal vessels. Findings related to narrowing of the central pulmonary arteries are volume loss, oligemia, and mosaic attenuation of the affected lung segments. Intraluminal thromboemboli may form. Venous narrowing and obstruction may cause mosaic attenuation or other parenchymal findings typical of edema, such as air space opacities and interlobular septal thickening. If the superior vena cava is affected, venous collaterals always form.[24]

FIGURE 4.11 — Fibrosing Mediastinitis

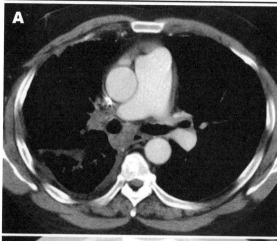

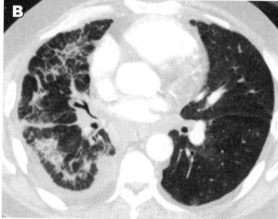

Dilatation of the main pulmonary artery and right mediastinal adenopathy *(A)*. Asymmetric pulmonary edema in the right lung *(B)*.

Pulmonary Veno-occlusive Disease

Pulmonary veno-occlusive disease is a rare idiopathic cause of PH that is characterized by obliterative lesions in the small proximal pulmonary veins. Clinically, the disease is similar to PAH, but because most of the resistance to pulmonary blood flow is distal to the pulmonary capillary bed. As a result, pulmonary capillary pressure is often elevated and pulmonary edema can occur despite normal or low left atrial and left ventricular end-diastolic pressure. Differentiation from PAH has important clinical implications because PAH-specific medications are ineffective and can increase pulmonary edema formation. Several findings on chest CT can help distinguish PVOD from PAH (**Figure 4.12**). In addition to the typical findings of PH, the combination of pulmonary edema and PH without plexiform arteriopathy in a child or young adult is highly suggestive of veno-occlusive disease.[3,25] Additional findings that may be present are ground glass opacities (often centrilobular), interlobular septal thickening (usually subpleural), well-defined lung nodules, mediastinal lymphadenopathy, and pleural and pericardial effusions.[26] The pulmonary veins should not be enlarged.

Capillary Hemangiomatosis

Frequently misdiagnosed, capillary hemangiomatosis has several CT findings that differentiate it from other forms of PH (**Figure 4.13**). In addition to main pulmonary artery enlargement, diffuse centrilobular ground glass nodules are a key feature found in most patients, and hemorrhagic pleural effusions are present in up to 25% of cases. More sporadic findings include interlobular septal thickening, mediastinal lymphadenopathy, and right heart chamber enlargement.[25]

Left-Sided Cardiac Disease

Transmission of elevated left heart pressure via left-sided ventricular or valvular cardiac disease is the most common cause of PH. Symmetric smooth interlobular septal thickening indicates pulmonary venous hypertension. Aortic valve calcification and left ventricular myocardial thickening suggests aortic stenosis. The mitral valve is difficult to assess without EKG-gating, although left atrial chamber enlargement with a calcified wall can be seen in mitral stenosis. A left atrial mass obstructing pulmonary venous return, such as a myxoma, can also cause PH.

Key Points

- General findings of PH on CT, regardless of etiology, are enlargement of the main pulmonary artery, pruning of the pulmonary arterial tree, right ventricular hypertrophy, and right atrial and ventricular enlargement.
- The combination of main pulmonary artery diameter >29 mm and a ratio of main pulmonary artery diameter to ascending aorta diameter >1 has high positive predictive value for PH, but their absence does not exclude the diagnosis.
- Mosaic attenuation is the main parenchymal change associated with PH. Regional variations in perfusion result in sharply demarcated areas of normal and low attenuation on CT.
- One advantage of CT is its ability to determine an underlying cause of PH in certain cases.
- Chronic pulmonary emboli can appear as eccentric filling defects or intraluminal bands or webs on CT angiography.
- In pulmonary fibrosis, the main pulmonary artery enlarges independently of pulmonary artery pressures. Measurement of main pulmonary artery diameter and its ratio with the ascending aorta is unreliable.

FIGURE 4.12 — Pulmonary Veno-occlusive Disease

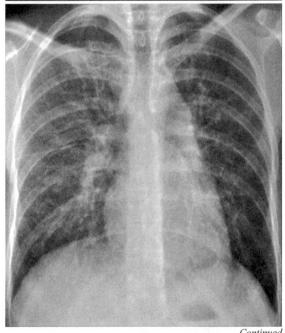

Continued

REFERENCES

1. Tan RT, Kuzo R, Goodman LR, et al. Utility of CT scan evaluation for predicting pulmonary hypertension in patients with parenchymal lung disease. Medical College of Wisconsin Lung Transplant Group. *Chest*. 1998;113(5):1250-1256.

2. NgCS, Wells AU, Padley SP. A CT sign of chronic pulmonary arterial hypertension: the ratio of main pulmonary artery to aortic diameter. *J Thorac Imaging*. 1999;14(4):270-278.

3. Grosse C, Grosse A. CT findings in diseases associated with pulmonary hypertension: a current review. *Radiographics*. 2010;30(7):1743-1777.

4. Frazier AA, Burke AP. The imaging of pulmonary hypertension. *Semin Ultrasound CT MR*. 2012;33(6):535-551.

FIGURE 4.12 — *Continued*

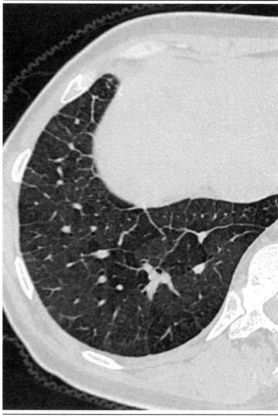

Chest x-ray showing dilatation of the main pulmonary artery and pulmonary edema in a patient with pulmonary veno-occlusive disease. Subpleural septal thickening is seen on chest CT.

5. Raymond RJ, Hinderliter AL, Willis PW, et al. Echocardio-graphic predictors of adverse outcomes in primary pulmonary hypertension. *J Am Coll Cardiol.* 2002;39(7):1214-1219.

6. Truong QA, Massaro JM, Rogers IS, et al. Reference values for normal pulmonary artery dimensions by noncontrast cardiac computed tomography: the Framingham Heart Study. *Circ Cardiovasc Imaging.* 2012;5(10):147-154.

FIGURE 4.13 — Capillary Hemangiomatosis

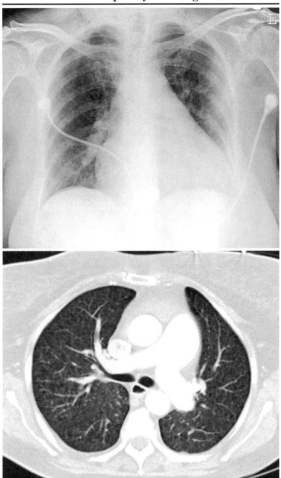

Continued

7. Castañer E, Gallardo X, Ballesteros E, et al. CT diagnosis of chronic pulmonary thromboembolism. *Radiographics*. 2009;29(1):31-50.

8. Rossi A, Attinà D, Borgonovi A, et al. Evaluation of mosaic pattern areas in HRCT with Min-IP reconstructions in patients with pulmonary hypertension: could this evaluation replace lung perfusion scintigraphy? *Eur J Radiol*. 2012;81(1):e1-6.

FIGURE 4.13 — *Continued*

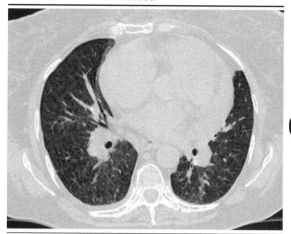

Dilatation of the main pulmonary artery and centrilobular ground glass nodules.

9. Auger WR, Fedullo PF, Moser KM, Buchbinder M, Peterson KL. Chronic major-vessel thromboembolic pulmonary artery obstruction: appearance at angiography. *Radiology*. 1992;182(2):393-398.

10. Remy-Jardin M, Duhamel A, Deken V, et al. Systemic collateral supply in patients with chronic thromboembolic and primary pulmonary hypertension: assessment with multi-detector row helical CT angiography. *Radiology*. 2005;235(1):274-281.

11. Sherrick AD, Swensen SJ, Hartman TE. Mosaic pattern of lung attenuation on CT scans: frequency among patients with pulmonary artery hypertension of different causes. *AJR Am J Roentgenol*. 1997;169(1):79-82.

12. Galiè N, Torbicki A, Barst R, et al. Guidelines on diagnosis and treatment of pulmonary arterial hypertension. The Task Force on Diagnosis and Treatment of Pulmonary Arterial Hypertension of the European Society of Cardiology. *Eur Heart J*. 2004;25(24):2243-2278.

13. van der Hulst AE, Roest AA, Westenberg JJ, Kroft LJ, de Roos A. Cardiac MRI in postoperative congenital heart disease patients. *J Magn Reson Imaging*. 2012;36(3):511-528.

14. Rajiah P, Kanne JP. Cardiac MRI: Part 1, cardiovascular shunts. *AJR Am J Roentgenol*.2011;197(4):W603-W620.

15. Galiè N, Hoeper MM, Humbert M, et al. Guidelines for the diagnosis and treatment of pulmonary hypertension. *Eur Respir J.* 2009;34(6):1219-1263.

16. Lettieri CJ, Nathan SD, Barnett SD, Ahmad S, Shorr AF. Prevalence and outcomes of pulmonary arterial hypertension in advanced idiopathic pulmonary fibrosis. *Chest.* 2006;129(3):745-752.

17. Zisman DA, Karlamangla AS, Ross DJ, et al. High-resolution chest CT findings do not predict the presence of pulmonary hypertension in advanced idiopathic pulmonary fibrosis. *Chest.* 2007;132(3):773-779.

18. Devaraj A, Wells AU, Meister MG, Corte TJ, Hansell DM. The effect of diffuse pulmonary fibrosis on the reliability of CT signs of pulmonary hypertension. *Radiology.* 2008;249(3):1042-1049.

19. Shujaat A, Bajwa AA, Cury JD. Pulmonary hypertension secondary to COPD. *Pulm Med.* 2012;2012:203952.

20. Le Pavec J, Lorillon G, Jaïs X, et al. Pulmonary Langerhans cell histiocytosis-associated pulmonary hypertension: clinical characteristics and impact of pulmonary arterial hypertension therapies. *Chest.* 2012;142(5):1150-1157.

21. Galvin JR, Franks TJ. Smoking-related lung disease. *J Thorac Imaging.* 2009;24(4):274-284.

22. McAdams HP, Erasmus J, Crockett R, et al. The hepatopulmonary syndrome: radiologic findings in 10 patients. *AJR Am J Roentgenol.* 1996;166(6):1379-1385.

23. Sherrick AD, Brown LR, Harms GF, Myers JL. The radiographic findings of fibrosing mediastinitis. *Chest.* 1994;106(2): 484-489.

24. Rossi SE, McAdams HP, Rosado-de-Christenson ML, et al. Fibrosing mediastinitis. *Radiographics.* 2001;21(3):737-757.

25. Frazier AA, Franks TJ, Mohammed TL, et al. From the Archives of the AFIP: pulmonary veno-occlusive disease and pulmonary capillary hemangiomatosis. *Radiographics.* 2007;27(3):867-882.

26. Resten A, Maitre S, Humbert M, et al. Pulmonary hypertension: CT of the chest in pulmonary venoocclusive disease. *AJR Am J Roentgenol.* 2004;183(1):65-70.

5

Approach to the Patient With Pulmonary Hypertension

by James R. Klinger, MD

Once the diagnosis of PH has been confirmed (see *Chapter 3*), the next step is to determine how it should be managed. This decision is centered on the type of PH that the patient has. The overall task of the clinician is presented in **Figure 5.1**. As can be seen from this diagram, clinical classification of PH into one of the five groups of PH described by the WHO determines which abnormalities may be responsible for the elevation in PAP and what therapies or procedures should be considered.

Assignment to one of the five WHO PH groups starts the patient and practitioner down distinctly different therapeutic pathways. Misclassification not only prevents the patient from receiving proper therapy but can result in the patient receiving expensive therapies that are not needed or in some cases, therapies that can significantly worsen the underlying condition. Once the patient's PH is properly classified, a variety of factors, including disease severity, rate of disease progression, and the patient's ability to manage a specific treatment, need to be considered, as discussed below.

Treatment Approach for Pulmonary Hypertension in WHO Group 1

Patients diagnosed with WHO Group 1 PAH have a progressive disease that often results in marked debilitation and death. As such, they require aggressive medical therapy and careful follow-up to assess response to treatment. Treatment guidelines and algorithms have been

FIGURE 5.1 — General Schematic Showing Overall Approach to a Patient With Elevated PAP

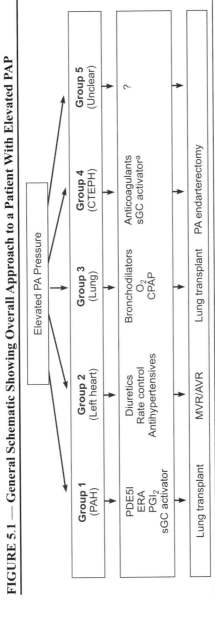

Group 1 (PAH)	Group 2 (Left heart)	Group 3 (Lung)	Group 4 (CTEPH)	Group 5 (Unclear)
PDE5I ERA PGI₂ sGC activator	Diuretics Rate control Antihypertensives	Bronchodilators O₂ CPAP	Anticoagulants sGC activator[a]	?
Lung transplant	MVR/AVR	Lung transplant	PA endarterectomy	

Elevated PA Pressure

[a] sGC activators are indicated for patients who are not candidates for PA endarterectomy or have PAH after endarterectomy.

The first step is to determine which of the five groups of pulmonary hypertensive disease the patient has (*top row*). The importance of making the proper diagnosis is demonstrated by the differences in medical therapies that should be used (*middle row*) and what surgical interventions are indicated if the patient has advanced disease or if medical therapy fails (*bottom row*).

developed by several professional societies including the 5th WHO Symposium on Pulmonary Hypertension, the American College of Chest Physicians, and the Joint Task Force of the European Society of Cardiology (ESC) and European Respiratory Society (ERS).[1-3] The most recent 2015 treatment guidelines are from ESC/ERS and are presented in **Figure 5.2**.[3] Their recommendations for efficacy of drugs, drug combinations, and sequential drug combinations for PAH are contained in **Tables 5.1**, **5.2**, and **5.3**.[3] Treatment guidelines for Group 1 PAH are based on three general principles:

1. Patients who demonstrate a significant acute pulmonary vasodilator response should be managed initially with CCBs instead of PAH-specific medications.
2. The most efficacious treatment for PAH is continuous intravenous prostacyclin infusion.
3. Patients with more severe or more rapidly progressive disease should be given more aggressive therapy.

These principles have been arrived at in large part by expert opinion as insufficient clinical data are available to make these recommendations on scientific grounds. In many cases, conclusions drawn about the efficacy of medications or management approaches are based on comparison of a given treatment to historical controls when PAH-specific therapies were not available. In particular, there has been a paucity of adequately controlled and sufficiently powered randomized controlled trials that examine the efficacy of one type of medication vs another. It is also unclear how efficacy should be measured. The primary outcome variable for the great majority of studies that led to the approval of currently available PAH therapies was the placebo-corrected change in 6MWD after 12 to 16 weeks of therapy. Most of these studies had secondary outcome measures showing improvement in WHO functional class, delay in the time for clinical worsening, and modest improvements in pulmonary

FIGURE 5.2 — 2015 ESC/ERS: Evidence-Based Treatment Algorithm for PAH Patients (Group 1 Only)

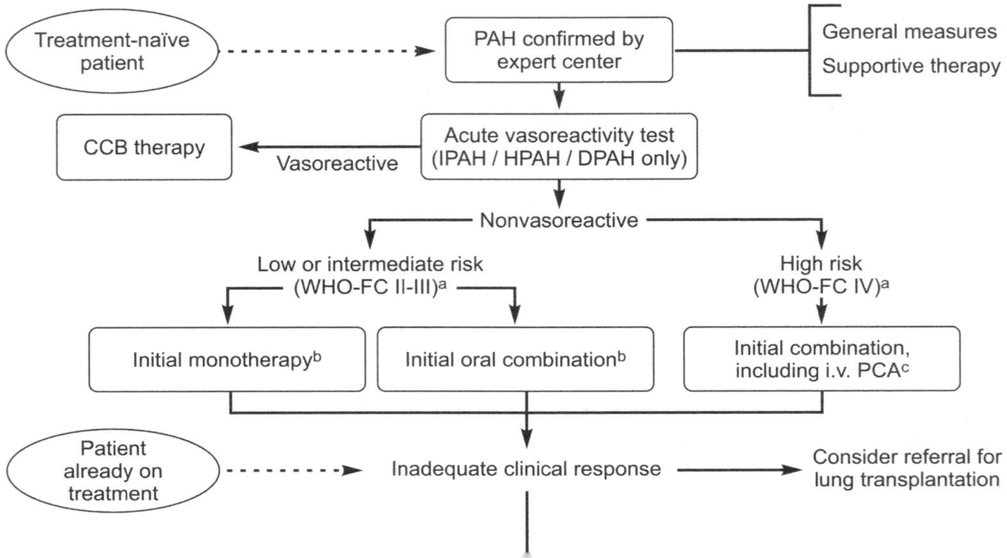

Treatment-naïve patient

PAH confirmed by expert center

General measures
Supportive therapy

Acute vasoreactivity test (IPAH / HPAH / DPAH only)

Vasoreactive

CCB therapy

Nonvasoreactive

Low or intermediate risk (WHO-FC II-III)[a]

High risk (WHO-FC IV)[a]

Initial monotherapy[b]

Initial oral combination[b]

Initial combination, including i.v. PCA[c]

Inadequate clinical response

Patient already on treatment

Consider referral for lung transplantation

102

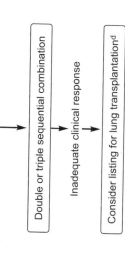

Double or triple sequential combination

Inadequate clinical response

Consider listing for lung transplantation[d]

[a] Some WHO-FC III patients may be considered high risk.

[b] Initial combination with ambrisentan plus tadalafil has proven to be superior to initial monotherapy with ambrisentan or tadalafil in delaying clinical failure.

[c] Intravenous epoprostenol should be prioritized as it has reduced the 3-months rate for mortality in high-risk PAH patients also as monotherapy.

[d] Consider also balloon atrial septostomy.

Galiè N, et al; Authors/Task Force Members. [published online ahead of print August 29, 2015]. *Eur Heart J.* doi: 10.1093/eurheartj/ehv317.

TABLE 5.1 — 2015 ESC/ERS: Recommendations for Efficacy of Drug Monotherapy for PAH (Group 1) According to WHO Functional Class

Measure/Treatment		Class[a]-Level[b]					
		WHO-FC II		WHO-FC III		WHO-FC IV	
Calcium channel blockers		I	C[c]	I	C[c]	—	—
Endothelin receptor antagonists	Ambrisentan	I	A	I	A	IIb	C
	Bosentan	I	A	I	A	IIb	C
	Macitentan[d]	I	B	I	B	IIb	C
Phosphodiesterase type-5 inhibitors	Sildenafil	I	A	I	A	IIb	C
	Tadalafil	I	B	I	B	IIb	C
	Vardenafil[e]	IIb	B	IIb	B	IIb	C
Guanylate cyclase stimulators	Riociguat	I	B	I	B	IIb	C
Prostacyclin analogues	Epoprostenol Intravenous[d]	—	—	I	A	I	A
	Iloprost Inhaled	—	—	I	B	IIb	C
	Iloprost Intravenous[e]	—	—	IIa	C	IIb	C

Treprostinil	Subcutaneous	—	—	I	B	IIb	C
	Inhaled[e]	—	—	I	B	IIb	C
	Intravenous[f]	—	—	IIa	C	IIb	C
	Oral[e]	—	—	IIb	B	—	—
Beraprost[e]		—	—	IIb	B	—	—
IP receptor agonists	Selexipag	Oral[e]	I	B	I	B	—	—

Sequence is by pharmacological group, by rating, and by alphabetical order.

[a] Class of recommendation.

[b] Level of evidence.

[c] Only in responders to acute vasoreactivity tests: class I (idiopathic PAH, heritable PAH, and PAH due to drugs); class IIa (conditions associated with PAH).

[d] Time to clinical worsening as primary endpoint in RCTs or drugs with demonstrated reduction in all-cause mortality.

[e] This drug is not approved by the EMA at the time of publication of these guidelines.

[f] In patients not tolerating the subcutaneous form.

Galiè N, et al; Authors/Task Force Members. [published online ahead of print August 29, 2015]. *Eur Heart J.* doi: 10.1093/eurheartj/ehv317.

5

105

TABLE 5.2 — 2015 ESC/ERS: Recommendations for Efficacy of Initial Drug Combination Therapy for PAH (Group 1) According to WHO Functional Class

Measure/Treatment	Class[a]-Level[b]					
	WHO-FC II		WHO-FC III		WHO-FC IV	
	I	B	I	B	IIb	C
Ambrisentan + tadalafil[d]	IIa	C	IIa	B	IIa	C
Other ERA + PDE5I	IIa	C	IIa	C	IIa	C
Bosentan + sildenafil + i.v. epoprostenol	—	—	IIa	C	IIa	C
Bosentan + i.v. epoprostenol	—	—	IIa	C	IIa	C
Other ERA or PDE5I + s.c. treprostinil			IIb	C	IIb	C
Other ERA or PDE5I + other i.v. prostacyclin analogues			IIb	C	IIb	C

Sequence is by rating.

[a] Class of recommendation.

[b] Level of evidence.

[c] Only in responders to acute vasoreactivity tests: class I (idiopathic PAH, heritable PAH, and PAH due to drugs); class IIa (conditions associated with PAH).

[d] Time to clinical failure as primary endpoint in RCTs or drugs with demonstrated reduction in all-cause mortality (prospectively defined).

Galiè N, et al; Authors/Task Force Members. [published online ahead of print August 29, 2015]. *Eur Heart J.* doi: 10.1093/eurheartj/ehv317.

hemodynamics. However, it is unclear if any of these outcome variables can be used to assess the efficacy of PAH therapies.

For example, a recent analysis has shown that the delay in clinical worsening observed in many studies of PAH therapies cannot be explained by improvements in 6MWD or PAP.[4] It is also unclear if improvement in any variable during the initial 12 to 16 weeks of therapy correlates with long-term responses beyond the first year of therapy. These issues were recently addressed in a long-term event driven study of the endothelin receptor antagonist (ERA) macitentan vs placebo given to WHO Group 1 patients in functional class II-III.[5] Approximately half of the patients were taking a phosphodiesterase type-5 inhibitor (PDE5I) at time of enrollment and continued to take it throughout the study. The other half of the study cohort was treatment naïve. This study was able to demonstrate that macitentan was more effective than placebo at preventing the occurrence of clinical worsening defined as a composite endpoint of death, hospitalization, lung transplantation, or initiation of intravenous prostacyclin therapy over a mean treatment duration of nearly 2 years.[5]

This study is important in that it was the first that was specifically designed to evaluate the efficacy of extended PAH therapy at slowing clinical disease progression and the first to demonstrate that a specific therapy (macitentan) was effective at doing so. Although other therapies currently available for PAH have not been examined in the same manner, their effect on other measures of efficacy, such as improvement in 6MWD, functional class, and pulmonary hemodynamics, is similar to that achieved with macitentan. Therefore, it is quite possible that these agents would have similar effects on delaying disease progression if studied in the same manner.

Current treatment guidelines recommend that before starting treatment, patients with Group 1 PAH first undergo testing to determine if they have a

TABLE 5.3 — 2015 ESC/ERS: Recommendations for Efficacy of Sequential Drug Combination Therapy for PAH (Group 1) According to WHO Functional Class

Measure/Treatment	Class[a]-Level[b]					
	WHO-FC II		WHO-FC III		WHO-FC IV	
Macitentan added to sildenafil[c]	I	B	I	B	IIa	C
Riociguat added to bosentan	I	B	I	B	IIa	C
Selexipag[d] added to ERA and/or PDE5I[c]	I	B	I	B	IIa	C
Sildenafil added to epoprostenol	—	—	I	B	IIa	B
Treprostinil inhaled added to sildenafil or bosentan	IIa	B	IIa	B	IIa	C
Iloprost inhaled added to bosentan	IIb	B	IIb	B	IIb	C
Tadalafil added to bosentan	IIa	C	IIa	C	IIa	C
Ambrisentan added to sildenafil	IIb	C	IIb	C	IIb	C
Bosentan added to epoprostenol	—	—	IIb	C	IIb	C
Bosentan added to sildenafil	IIb	C	IIb	C	IIb	C
Sildenafil added to bosentan	IIb	C	IIb	C	IIb	C

Other double combinations	IIb	C	IIb	C	IIb	C
Other triple combinations	IIb	C	IIb	C	IIb	C
Riociguat added to sildenafil or other PDE5I	III	B	III	B	III	B

Sequence is by rating and by alphabetical order.

[a] Class of recommendation.

[b] Level of evidence.

[c] Time to clinical worsening as primary endpoint in RCTs or drugs with demonstrated reduction in all-cause mortality (prospectively defined).

[d] This drug was not approved by the EMA at the time of publication of these guidelines.

Galiè N, et al; Authors/Task Force Members. [published online ahead of print August 29, 2015]. *Eur Heart J*. doi: 10.1093/eurheartj/ehv317.

significant pulmonary vasodilator response.[1,2] This is usually done by measuring the acute change in mean PA pressure to inhaled NO, intravenous prostacyclin, or adenosine during RHC. A fall in mean PAP $\geq$10 mm Hg from baseline to a mean PAP $\leq$40 mm Hg without any decrease in cardiac output indicates a positive response, and these patients should be given a trial of CCBs.[1,2]

These criteria are based on the rationale that elevation of PAP is due to either an increase in pulmonary vascular smooth muscle contraction (increased pulmonary vascular tone) or to narrowing of the pulmonary vascular lumen caused by the abnormal growth of pulmonary vascular cells (pulmonary vascular remodeling). The former responds well to CCBs, whereas the latter does not. Patients who drop their mPAP >10 mm Hg but still have an mPAP >40 mm Hg after vasodilator challenge are felt to have a combination of both increased pulmonary vascular tone and pulmonary vascular remodeling. When the mPAP after vasodilator challenge is >40 mm Hg, a sizable component of the increased PAP can be attributed to pulmonary vascular remodeling. In these patients, CCBs would not be expected to have long-term efficacy.

Limited studies have shown that PAH patients with a positive pulmonary vasodilator response do well when treated with CCBs alone. In one study, PAH patients with a positive vasodilator response had a 5-year survival of 94% when treated with CCBs compared with 55% in patients with a negative pulmonary vasodilator response.[6] However, only about 12% of PAH patients have a positive pulmonary vasodilator response and approximately half of those who respond demonstrate long-term improvement with CCBs alone.[7] Thus, the number of PAH patients who have a sustained beneficial response to CCBs is quite small. Considering that the great majority of patients with a pulmonary vasodilator response have IPAH, HPAH, or APAH associated with the use of anorectic drugs, many experts feel that acute vasodilator testing is unwarranted in patients with other forms of PAH such as PAH associated with connective tissue disease, portal hypertension, or HIV infection.[3]

For the majority of PAH patients who do not exhibit an acute vasodilator response, recommendations for initial treatment are based on risk stratification. Guidelines for assessing disease severity and risk of disease progression are shown in **Table 5.4**. Patients in WHO functional class I or II with gradual onset of symptoms, no clinical signs of right heart failure, 6MWD >440 meters, normal or mildly elevated BNP or NT-BNP, and normal RV function and cardiac output at rest are considered to have mild to moderate disease and are at low risk for rapid deterioration. Those with worse symptoms, signs of right heart failure, decreased functional capacity, and poor right ventricular function are considered to have more advanced disease and to be at greater risk of worsening.

Current treatment guidelines recommend treating functional class II or III patients who are in the low or intermediate risk category with a PDE5I or ERA.[1,2] The greater the number of poor prognostic indicators, the more the clinician should consider using a prostacyclin infusion as initial therapy. This approach allows patients with less advanced disease the opportunity to respond to orally active agents and prevents patients from taking on the burden and expense of continuous intravenous or subcutaneous infusion. Inherent in these recommendations is the need for careful monitoring of disease progression and patient response to therapy. Patients are usually seen every 4 to 8 weeks during initial therapy until a favorable response is achieved and then every 3 months afterwards. Patients who do not respond to initial therapy within 3 months are given additional therapies until one or a combination of therapies achieves the desired effect or until all available therapies have been tried.

The definition of an adequate clinical response remains unclear, but most experts believe that patients should improve their functional class by at least one category (eg, from functional class III to II) or achieve

TABLE 5.4 — 2015 ESC/ERS: Risk Assessment in PAH

Determinants of Prognosis[a] (estimated 1-y mortality)	Low Risk <5%	Intermediate Risk 5%-10%	High Risk >10%
Clinical signs of right heart failure	Absent	Absent	Present
Progression of symptoms	No	Slow	Rapid
Syncope	No	Occasional syncope[b]	Repeated syncope[c]
WHO functional class	I, II	III	IV
6MWD	>440 m	165-440 m	<165 m
Cardiopulmonary exercise testing	Peak VO$_2$ >15 mL/min/kg (>65% predicted) VE/VCO$_2$ slope <36	Peak VO$_2$ 11-15 mL/min/kg (35%-65% predicted) VE/VCO$_2$ slope 36-44.9	Peak VO$_2$ <11 mL/min/kg (<35% predicted) VE/VCO$_2$ ≥45
NT-proBNP plasma levels	BNP <50 ng/L NT-proBNP <300 ng/mL	BNP 50-300 ng/L NT-proBNP 300-1400 ng/L	BNP >300 ng/L NT-proBNP >1400 ng/L

Imaging (echocardiography, CMR imaging)	RA area <18 cm^2 No pericardial effusion	RA area 18-26 cm^2 No or minimal pericardial effusion	RA area >26 cm^2 Pericardial effusion
Hemodynamics	RAP <8 mm Hg CI ≥2.5 L/min/m^2 SvO$_2$ >65%	RAP 8-14 mm Hg CI 2.0-2.4 L/min/m^2 SvO$_2$ 60%-65%	RAP >14 mm Hg CI <2.0 L/min/m^2 SvO$_2$ <60%

[a] Most of the proposed variables and cut-off values are based on expert opinion. They may provide prognostic information and may be used to guide therapeutic decisions, but not necessarily apply to other forms of PAH. Furthermore, the use of approved therapies and their influence on the variables should be considered in the evaluation of the risk.

[b] Occasional syncope during brisk or heavy exercise, or occasional orthostatic syncope in an otherwise stable patient.

[c] Repeated episodes of syncope, even with little or regular physical activity.

Galiè N, et al; Authors/Task Force Members. [published online ahead of print August 29, 2015]. *Eur Heart J.* doi: 10.1093/eurheartj/ehv317.

a 6MWD and/or BNP level that is associated with low risk of disease progression or death (**Table 5.4** and **Figure 5.3**).[8] These treatment goals are not universally accepted and some practitioners will leave patients on their initial therapy, if they are at low or intermediate risk of disease progression as long as they do not deteriorate. There is general agreement, however, that patients who demonstrate disease progression manifesting as either worsening dyspnea, worsening

FIGURE 5.3 — Goal-Oriented Approach to Treatment of Pulmonary Hypertension

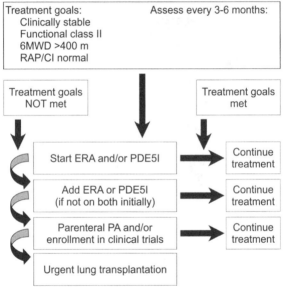

Rather than waiting for a patient's clinical status to deteriorate, this approach sets predetermined goals for the patient to achieve prior to starting therapy. Patients are assessed at the end of 3 to 6 months treatment with each therapy and if the clinical goals have not been met, additional therapy is given and the patient's status is reassessed in 3 to 6 months. Patients who fail to meet treatment goals despite maximal medical therapy are referred for lung transplant evaluation.

Modified from Hoeper MM, et al. *Eur Respir J.* 2005;26(5):858-863.

right ventricular function on echocardiogram, or a >10% decrease in 6MWD, be given additional medical therapy until an adequate trial of each of the presently available classes of PAH medications has been tried. When clinical assessment reveals conflicting information (eg, a patient whose 6MWD has improved but who has a rise in BNP and deterioration of RV function on echo), right heart catheterization can be helpful to determine if their PH has worsened.

For patients who present in WHO functional class IV or who are at high risk of deterioration (**Table 5.4**), most experts feel that continuous intravenous infusion of epoprostenol is the most efficacious therapy (**Figure 5.2**). The rationale for this opinion is discussed in greater detail in this book, but in part, centers on how intravenous prostacyclin therapy is administered. Unlike orally active PAH-specific therapies that are given at one or two fixed doses, the infusion rate of parenteral prostacyclins is continuously adjusted upward to the patient's maximally tolerated dose. During the first 3 to 6 months of therapy, patients may have their dose increased >10-fold. Thus, the efficacy of parenteral prostacyclin may be due in part to its individualized dosing regimen and/or its intravenous route of administration.

Regardless of the reason for its efficacy, intravenous epoprostenol is one of the few therapies that have been associated with reduced mortality during the first 12 weeks of therapy, although the study in which improved survival was observed was not placebo controlled and most patients had more advanced disease than those in studies of other PAH medications.[9] Unfortunately, the risks of infection and bleeding inherent with the need for a central venous catheter, along with the risk of sudden decompensation if the infusion is interrupted, makes this therapy the most challenging to administer. Inhaled and orally active prostacyclin therapies have also been developed and approved for treatment of PAH, but their clinical efficacy does not appear to be as robust as that of intravenous epoprostenol infusion.[10,11] Although their comparative ease of use may provide access to prostacyclin therapy for some patients who are incapable of managing continuous intravenous infusion, inhaled or oral prostacyclin therapy should not be considered to be the equivalent of intravenous prostacyclin therapy.

Due to the lack of properly controlled comparator trials that examine the relative efficacy of the presently available PAH treatments, it is not possible to determine if one type of therapy is actually more effective at treating PAH than any other or if a combination of therapies is better than treatment with a single agent. Randomized, placebo-controlled studies have demonstrated improvement in 6MWD, pulmonary hemodynamics, and/or time to clinical worsening with the addition of oral sildenafil to intravenous epoprostenol,[12] or the addition of inhaled treprostinil to patients on a steady dose of a PDE5I or an ERA.[11] or the addition of riociguat to patients on stable dose of an ERA or nonintravenous prostacyclin.[13] However, in each of these studies, it is unclear if the improved responses were due to the additive effects of combining two therapies or if patients in the trials were simply more responsive to the new therapy that was added to their background therapy.

A recently completed trial has attempted to determine the relative efficacy of combined vs monotherapy as initial treatment for PAH. The AMBITION trial reported results from 500 treatment-naïve PAH patients in functional class II or III who were randomized to initial treatment with tadalafil or ambrisentan or the combination of tadalafil and ambrisentan in a 1:1:2 pattern.

The primary endpoint of clinical failure defined as the first occurrence of death, hospitalization for worsening PAH, disease progression, or unsatisfactory long-term clinical response occurred in 18% of patients treated with the combination of tadalafil and ambrisentan and in 31% of the patients in the two monotherapy groups combined (hazard ratio for the combination-therapy group vs the pooled monotherapy group was 0.50 [95% CI, 0.35-0.72; *P*<0.001]) (**Figure 5.4**).[14] The difference in event rates between the combination and pooled monotherapy groups was driven primarily by a reduction in the rate of hospitalization for PAH which was 3 times greater in the pooled monotherapy group than it was in the combination-therapy group. After 24 weeks of treatment, patients in the combination-therapy group had a greater reduction from baseline in N-terminal pro-BNP (-67.2% vs -50.4%; *P*<0.001)

5

FIGURE 5.4 — AMBITION Trial: Kaplan–Meier Curves for the Probability of First Event of Clinical Failure

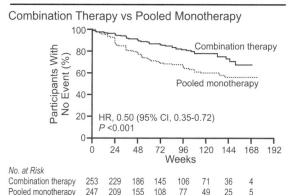

Combination Therapy vs Pooled Monotherapy

No. at Risk								
	0	24	48	72	96	120	144	168
Combination therapy	253	229	186	145	106	71	36	4
Pooled monotherapy	247	209	155	108	77	49	25	5

Time to first event of clinical failure defined as death from any cause, hospitalization for worsening PAH, disease progression, or unsatisfactory long-term clinical response in treatment-naïve patients with PAH who were given a combination of ambrisentan 10 mg daily plus tadalafil 40 mg daily compared with patients treated with either drug alone. Patients were randomized to treatment with ambrisentan, tadalafil, or ambrisentan + tadalafil in a 1:1:2 ratio. Data from patients given ambrisentan alone or tadalafil alone were combined (pooled monotherapy). The events rate for each treatment group were 34% for ambrisentan alone, 28% for tadalafil alone, 31% for the pooled monotherapy groups, and 18% for the combination of ambrisentan + tadalafil.

Galiè N, et al. *N Eng J Med*. 2015;373:834-844.

and a greater increase in 6MWD (median change from baseline, 49.0 m vs 23.8 m; $P<0.001$) than patients in the pooled monotherapy group, although there was no difference in the proportion of patients who improved or worsened by at least one functional class. Peripheral edema, headache, and nasal congestion occurred more often in the combination-therapy group than in either of the monotherapy groups, but the rate of discontinuation of study drug and serious adverse events were similar in all three groups. These results support the growing body of evidence that PAH-specific therapies may be more effective at improving outcomes when used in combination. Although additional studies may be needed to determine if switching from one therapy to another when a patient worsens or fails to improve is as effective as up-front combination therapy, it seems reasonable to consider the combination of a PDE5I and ERA as initial treatment for patients with newly diagnosed PAH in functional class II or III, particularly if they are at intermediate risk of disease progression (**Figure 5**.2 and **Table 5**.4).

For patients who are not improving on a given therapy, most PH experts favor adding new therapies rather than switching from one to another.[2] This approach allows for examining patient response to each drug class as well as the response to combination therapy. When a patient who has not responded to one therapy improves following the addition of another, it can be difficult to determine if both medications should be continued or if the initial medication or medications should be stopped. Due to our limited ability to determine which patients are likely to benefit from which drugs, most practitioners experienced in PAH opt to continue multiple therapies knowing that if the patient deteriorates when one is stopped, it may be difficult to reverse their decline by restarting the discontinued drug.

Patients with PAH in WHO functional class I represent a unique challenge. Few patients with asymptomatic PAH have been included in clinical trials and it is not clear whether treatment of PAH at an early stage can prevent disease progression. In the one study that addressed the question of treatment for early stage PAH, the primary outcome measure (change in 6MWD test from baseline) was not met.[15] However, there was a strong trend in favor of patients who received the study drug (bosentan) and a significant improvement in secondary outcome measures including time to clinical worsening vs patients given placebo. Recently published treatment guidelines recommend careful follow-up of functional class I PAH patients, but no treatment.[1] However, consideration for treatment should be given to WHO functional class I patients who have other adverse prognostic indicators outlined in **Table 5**.4.

Approach to Non-Group 1 Pulmonary Hypertension

All of the presently approved therapies for PH, with the exception of riociguat, are indicated only for the treatment of WHO Group 1. Riociguat is indicated for treatment of both WHO Group 1 and WHO Group 4—CTEPH (see *Chapter 11* for treatment of Group 4). Thus, there are no approved PH therapies for treatment of WHO Groups 2, 3, or 5. However, Groups 2 and 3 represent the vast majority of patients with PH and it can often be challenging to differentiate patients with Group 1 vs Group 2 or 3 PH. In particular, left-sided heart disease is the most common cause of elevated PAP. In some studies, as much as three fourths of all cases of PH identified on echocardiogram were ultimately found to be due to left ventricular dysfunction or left-sided valvular heart disease.[16]

The use of pulmonary vasodilator therapies is not recommended in these patients for several reasons. First, patients with pulmonary venous pressures measured by PCWP or LVEDP >15 have been excluded from nearly all clinical trials of presently available medications leaving insufficient data to determine if these medications are at all helpful in this form of PH. Second, increasing blood flow through the pulmonary circulation via administration of pulmonary vasodilators will increase left-sided filling pressures thereby aggravating left-sided heart failure. Finally, a recently completed randomized controlled trial of sildenafil for the treatment of PH associated with left ventricular diastolic dysfunction was found to be negative.[17]

The primary tenant of withholding pulmonary vasodilators from patients with left-sided heart disease is that the elevation of PAP in these patients is not due to pulmonary vasoconstriction or to vascular remodeling, but to elevated pulmonary venous pressure. However, in many patients with long-standing pulmonary venous pressure, the transpulmonary gradient, defined as the difference between mean PAP and PCWP, can become elevated. This increase in pulmonary vascular resistance may protect the left heart from excessive preload. Decreasing the transpulmonary gradient in these patients can lead to increased dyspnea or pulmonary edema. Due to the large number of patients with Group 2 PH and the poor prognosis of PH associated with left heart disease, it has become increasingly difficult not to offer these patients any of the numerous medications that have been developed for PAH. However, without any data to support their use in this population of patients, the high cost and potential adverse events of presently approved PAH drugs precludes their use in these patients.

PH occurs commonly in patients with chronic lung disease and often leads to right ventricular failure otherwise known as cor pulmonale. While hypoxia and hypoxemia are well-known causes of increased pulmonary vascular tone, the etiology of PH associated with lung disease is more complex than oxygen insufficiency. Many of the abnormalities in vascular growth factors seen in Group 1 PAH including decreased expression of eNOS and increased expression of interleukin-6 are seen in cigarette smokers and patients with emphysema.[18,19] Patients with obstructive sleep apnea often have systemic hypertension, LV diastolic, or systolic dysfunction, in addition to recurrent hypoxemia. Finally, patients with pulmonary fibrosis or emphysema have considerable destruction of lung parenchyma and reduced number of pulmonary vessels that may contribute to the increase in PVR. Therefore, treatment of PH in these patients is usually not effective, and management should be directed toward treatment of their underlying disease.

Adequate oxygenation can be very important in this setting. Optimal and minimal levels of arterial oxygen saturation have not been well studied in PAH, but most guidelines recommend maintaining arterial O_2 saturation at $\geq$92%. It should be noted, however, that the individual pulmonary vasoconstrictive response to hypoxia is quite variable with some patients exhibiting sensitivity to even mild hypoxia. This is particularly true in patients with hypercapnea as elevated pCO_2 tension and decreased pH can enhance the hypoxic pulmonary vasoconstriction response.[20] In the catheterization lab, it is often worthwhile to determine if PAP decreases on 100% O_2 saturation. Although most patients are not considered for supplemental O_2 until arterial saturation is <88%, it should be noted that Medicare guidelines provide for supplemental O_2 when arterial saturation is <92% in patients with PH or cor pulmonale. Even in patients with systemic O_2 saturation >92% on room air, care should be taken to exclude intermittent hypoxia as may occur in sleep disordered breathing.

The use of PAH-specific therapies in patients with PH that is attributable to lung disease is not recommended. Similar to Group 2 PH, PAH-specific therapies have not been well studied in Group 3 patients and in the few small studies that have been done, no improvement was seen in functional capacity or dyspnea. Furthermore, both sildenafil and bosentan have been shown to cause mild worsening of oxygenation in patients with COPD.[21,22] Finally, both sildenafil and bosentan have been studied in pulmonary fibrosis patients and found to be of little benefit.[23-25]

Patients with Group 5 PH have a variety of pulmonary vascular diseases that are not well understood. These patients may be the least studied of all and treatment recommendations for this group have been difficult to come by due to the small number of patients and the lack of clinical data. Small, open-label studies have reported some success in PH associated with Langerhans histocytosis X and PH associated with sarcoidosis,[25-27] and it may be reasonable to consider PH in these patients especially when the degree of PH appears to be greater than would be expected from their lung disease alone. Randomized controlled studies of PAH-specific therapies in these patients are needed before better treatment recommendations can be made. Sildenafil was studied in patients with PH associated with sickle cell disease but was not found to be helpful and may have caused adverse effects.[28] Treatment of PH in sickle cell disease can be particularly challenging and most cases of PH in sickle cell patients do not have an elevated transpulmonary gradient. An approach to diagnosis and treatment of PH associated with sickle cell and guidelines to treating pulmonary vascular disease in sickle cell patients have recently been published.[29]

Management of patients with WHO Group 2, 3, or 5 PH represents a unique challenge. Most of the pulmonary vascular disease that occurs in these patients is the result of chronic disease processes that will not improve in response to PAH-specific medications. Even when PAH-specific medications result in a lowering of PAP or PVR, the underlying condition persists and often prevents the patient from experiencing any improvement in dyspnea or other symptoms. PAH-specific medications can also increase left ventricular filling pressures and worsen gas exchange thereby aggravating the patients underlying disease. In lack of any data suggesting clear benefit, the use of PAH-specific medications is not recommended for patients with these types of PH.

The decision not to treat PH in this situation is often met with discouragement and frustration, especially when the patient has few other treatment options and diagnostic studies consistently demonstrate increasing PAP and right heart failure. However, management for these patients should be directed at aggressive treatment of their underlying heart or lung disease and reassurance that adding expensive medications with potential adverse effects will not be helpful. When patients appear to have PH that is out of proportion to their underlying disease, it may be beneficial to refer the patient to a center that is experienced in the management of PAH. Many centers have developed specific approaches regarding when and to what extent PH should be treated in these patients. These centers are also often engaged in ongoing clinical trials that may help identify if there are subsets of WHO Group 2, 3, or 5 PH that may benefit from PAH-specific therapies in the future.

Key Points

- Proper diagnosis and classification of PH using the WHO classification scheme is essential to ensuring appropriate management.
- Patients with WHO Group 1 PAH with moderate disease and at low or intermediate risk of rapid deterioration should be considered for oral therapies. Those with advanced disease or at risk of rapid deterioration should be considered for parenteral prostacyclin infusion.
- Medical management of PAH patients requires close follow up. Patients who fail to improve in response to a class of PAH-specific drug should be given an additional drug class, usually in combination with their initial therapy. Recent studies suggest that up front combination with a PDE5I and ERA is more effective at preventing clinical failure than initial treatment with either agent alone.

- PH due to chronic heart and lung disease has not been shown to respond to PAH-specific medications. Patients with PH that appears to be out of proportion to their heart or lung disease may benefit from referral to a center experienced in the diagnosis and treatment of PAH.

REFERENCES

1. Taichman DB, Ornelas J, Chung L, et al. Pharmacologic therapy for pulmonary arterial hypertension in adults: CHEST guideline and expert panel report. *Chest*. 2014;146(2):449-475.

2. Galiè N, Corris PA, Frost A, et al. Updated treatment algorithm of pulmonary arterial hypertension. *J Am Coll Cardiol*. 2013;62(25 suppl):D60-D72.

3. Galiè N, Humbert M, Vachiery JL, et al; Authors/Task Force Members. 2015 ESC/ERS Guidelines for the diagnosis and treatment of pulmonary hypertension: The Joint Task Force for the Diagnosis and Treatment of Pulmonary Hypertension of the European Society of Cardiology (ESC) and the European Respiratory Society (ERS), Endorsed by: Association for European Paediatric and Congenital Cardiology (AEPC), International Society for Heart and Lung Transplantation (ISHLT). 2015 ESC/ERS guidelines for the diagnosis and treatment of pulmonary hypertension [published online ahead of print August 29, 2015]. *Eur Heart J*. 2015. doi: 10.1093/eurheartj/ehv317.

4. Ventetuolo CE, Gabler NB, Fritz JS, et al. Are hemodynamics surrogate end points in pulmonary arterial hypertension? *Circulation*. 2014;130(9):768-775.

5. Pulido T, Adzerikho I, Channick RN, et al; SERAPHIN Investigators. Macitentan and morbidity and mortality in pulmonary arterial hypertension. *N Engl J Med*. 2013;369(9):809-818.

6. Rich S, Kaufmann E, Levy PS. The effect of high doses of calcium-channel blockers on survival in primary pulmonary hypertension. *N Engl J Med*. 1992;327(2):76-81.

7. Sitbon O, Humbert M, Jaïs X, et al. Long-term response to calcium channel blockers in idiopathic pulmonary arterial hypertension. *Circulation*. 2005;111(23):3105-3111.

8. Hoeper MM, Markevych I, Spiekerkoetter E, Welte T, Niedermeyer J. Goal-oriented treatment and combination therapy for pulmonary arterial hypertension. *Eur Respir J*. 2005;26(5):858-863.

9. Barst RJ, Rubin LJ, Long WA, et al. A comparison of continuous intravenous epoprostenol (prostacyclin) with conventional therapy for primary pulmonary hypertension. The Primary Pulmonary Hypertension Study Group. *N Engl J Med.* 1996;334:296-302.

10. Simonneau G, Barst RJ, Galie N, et al; Treprostinil Study Group. Continuous subcutaneous infusion of treprostinil, a prostacyclin analogue, in patients with pulmonary arterial hypertension: a double-blind, randomized, placebo-controlled trial. *Am J Respir Crit Care Med.* 2002;165(6):800-804.

11. McLaughlin VV, Benza RL, Rubin LJ, et al. Addition of inhaled treprostinil to oral therapy for pulmonary arterial hypertension: a randomized controlled clinical trial. *J Am Coll Cardiol.* 2010;55:1915-1922.

12. Simonneau G, Rubin LJ, Galie N, et al. Addition of sildenafil to long-term intravenous epoprostenol therapy in patients with pulmonary arterial hypertension: a randomized trial. *Ann Intern Med.* 2008;149:521-530.

13. Ghofrani HA, Galiè N, Grimminger F, et al; PATENT-1 Study Group. Riociguat for the treatment of pulmonary arterial hypertension. *N Engl J Med.* 2013;369(4):330-340.

14. Galiè N, Barberà JA, Frost AE, et al; AMBITION Investigators. Initial use of ambrisentan plus tadalafil in pulmonary arterial hypertension. *N Engl J Med.* 2015;373(9):834-844.

15. Galiè N, Rubin Lj, Hoeper M, et al. Treatment of patients with mildly symptomatic pulmonary arterial hypertension with bosentan (EARLY study): a double-blind, randomised controlled trial. *Lancet.* 2008;371(9630):2093-2100.

16. Strange G, Playford D, Stewart S, et al. Pulmonary hypertension: prevalence and mortality in the Armadale echocardiography cohort. *Heart.* 2012;98(24):1805-1811.

17. Redfield MM, Chen HH, Borlaug BA, et al; RELAX Trial. Effect of phosphodiesterase-5 inhibition on exercise capacity and clinical status in heart failure with preserved ejection fraction: a randomized clinical trial. *JAMA.* 2013;309(12):1268-1277.

18. Barberà JA, Peinado VI, Santos S, Ramirez J, Roca J, Rodriguez-Roisin R. Reduced expression of endothelial nitric oxide synthase in pulmonary arteries of smokers. *Am J Respir Crit Care Med.* 2001;164(4):709-713.

19. Chaouat A, Savale L, Chouaid C, et al. Role for interleukin-6 in COPD-related pulmonary hypertension. *Chest.* 2009;136(3):678-687.

5

20. Rudolph AM, Yuan S. Response of the pulmonary vasculature to hypoxia and H+ ion concentration changes. *J Clin Invest*. 1966;45(3):399-411.

21. Stolz D, Rasch H, Linka A, et al. A randomised, controlled trial of bosentan in severe COPD. *Eur Respir J*. 2008;32(3):619-628.

22. Blanco I, Gimeno E, Munoz PA, et al. Hemodynamic and gas exchange effects of sildenafil in patients with chronic obstructive pulmonary disease and pulmonary hypertension. *Am J Respir Crit Care Med*. 2010;181(3):270-278.

23. Idiopathic Pulmonary Fibrosis Clinical Research Network; Zisman DA, Schwarz M, Anstrom KJ, Collard HR, Flaherty KR, Hunninghake GW. A controlled trial of sildenafil in advanced idiopathic pulmonary fibrosis. *N Engl J Med*. 2010;363(7):620-628.

24. Corte TJ, Keir GJ, Dimopoulos K, et al; BPHIT Study Group. Bosentan in pulmonary hypertension associated with fibrotic idiopathic interstitial pneumonia. *Am J Respir Crit Care Med*. 2014;190(2):208-217.

25. King TE Jr, Brown KK, Raghu G, et al. BUILD-3: a randomized, controlled trial of bosentan in idiopathic pulmonary fibrosis. *Am J Respir Crit Care Med*. 2011;184(1):92-99.

26. Le Pavec J, Lorillon G, Jaïs X, et al. Pulmonary Langerhans cell histiocytosis-associated pulmonary hypertension: clinical characteristics and impact of pulmonary arterial hypertension therapies. *Chest*. 2012;142(5):1150-1157.

27. Baughman RP, Culver DA, Cordova FC, et al. Bosentan for sarcoidosis-associated pulmonary hypertension: a double-blind placebo controlled randomized trial. *Chest*. 2014;145(4):810-817.

28. Barnett CF, Bonura EJ, Nathan SD, et al. Treatment of sarcoidosis-associated pulmonary hypertension. A two-center experience. *Chest*. 2009;135(6):1455-1461.

29. Machado RF, Barst RJ, Yovetich NA, et al; walk-PHaSST Investigators and Patients. Hospitalization for pain in patients with sickle cell disease treated with sildenafil for elevated TRV and low exercise capacity. *Blood*. 2011;118(4):855-864.

30. Klings ES, Machado RF, Barst RJ, et al; American Thoracic Society Ad Hoc Committee on Pulmonary Hypertension of Sickle Cell Disease. An official American Thoracic Society clinical practice guideline: diagnosis, risk stratification, and management of pulmonary hypertension of sickle cell disease. *Am J Respir Crit Care Med*. 2014;189(6):727-740.

6
Prostacyclin Therapy

by James R. Klinger, MD

Introduction

The approval of epoprostenol by the FDA in December of 1995 ushered in the era of prostacyclin treatment for PAH. It was the first drug to be developed and approved specifically for the treatment of PAH and remains a cornerstone of the therapeutic management of this disease. Intravenous prostacyclin therapy remains the only therapy that has demonstrated improved survival in a randomized clinical trial of PAH[1] and is widely considered to be the most efficacious treatment despite the development of more than a half dozen new PAH-specific medications since epoprostenol was first approved.

Development of Prostacyclin Therapy for PAH

Prostacyclin was discovered and first reported by Dr. John Vane's laboratory in 1976.[2] The first report describes "an unstable substance described as PG-X" that was derived from prostaglandins G_2 and H_2 and inhibited human platelet aggregation with a potency that was 30 times greater than PGE_1.[2] Later that year, the chemical structure was reported by Whittiker and colleagues,[3] and the term prostacyclin was suggested. Using the systematic chemical nomenclature of prostaglandins, the chemical structure of prostacyclin corresponds to PGI_2. Prostacyclin is synthesized from prostaglandin H_2 primarily by vascular endothelial cells[4,5] via prostaglandin synthase where it plays a vital role in counteracting the thrombotic and vasoconstrictive effects of thromboxane. The term prostacyclin refers to the endogenous prostaglandin isolated from animal tissues.

Epoprostenol refers to prostacyclin that has been chemically synthesized. Epoprostenol was developed and tested in animals by a team of investigators from the Wellcome Foundation headed by John Vane and fellow researchers Salvador Moncada, Ryszard Gryglewski, and Stuart Bunting shortly after the discovery of prostacyclin.[6] Epoprostenol would go on to be tested in humans and eventually was developed for commercial use as a medical therapeutic. In an effort to develop a prostacyclin-like compound that was more stable and thus better suited for in vivo testing and clinical development, the Vane team synthesized hundreds of prostacyclin analogues. For this work, Dr. Vane was awarded the Nobel Prize in Physiology and Medicine in 1982 and knighted by Queen Elizabeth in 1984.

In addition to its potent inhibitory effect on platelet aggregation, it was quickly realized that prostacyclin is a potent vasodilator, particularly in the pulmonary vascular bed where its effect was found to be sustained about 10-fold longer than PGE_1, the other known prostaglandin with vasodilator properties in mature animals.[7] It was also noted that the dilator response to prostacyclin was enhanced when PVR was increased and that prostacyclin had less effect on cardiac output and aortic pressure than PGE_1. Prostacyclin also has anti-inflammatory effects and has been shown to have antiproliferative effects on vascular endothelial and smooth muscle cells. These findings along with other studies showing that prostacyclin synthesis was decreased in PAH[8,9] suggested that prostacyclins may be particularly well suited for the treatment of pulmonary vascular disease and led to the development of several prostanoid therapies for PAH, including prostacyclin derivatives that can be delivered by subcutaneous infusion, inhalation, and even the oral route.

The biologic effects of prostacyclin and most of its analogues are mediated via the G-protein coupled prostaglandin I_2 receptor (IP_1). Ligand binding results in a conformational change in the receptor and activation of Gs which signals adenylyl cyclase to produce cAMP.[10] This raises intracellular cAMP levels that activate protein kinase A (PKA). PKA acts downstream by inhibiting myosin light-chain kinase, which leads to smooth muscle relaxation. Prostacyclin also binds to the adenylyl cyclase linked prostaglandin E receptor (EP). More recently, non-cAMP effects of prostacyclin have been demonstrated via binding to the intracellular receptor PPAR-gamma.[11] The relative binding affinities of the synthetic prostacyclin analogues for IP, EP, and PPAR-gamma varies between compounds and may be responsible for differences in biologic properties. As a result, there may be significant differences in biologic effects between the different prostacyclin analogues that have been developed for treatment of PAH.

Presently, three prostacyclin analogues—epoprostenol, treprostinil, and iloprost—are available for the treatment of PAH in the United States (**Table 6.1**). Intravenous epoprostenol, like prostacyclin, has an extremely short half-life and is unstable at room temperatures, resulting in the need for continuous infusion therapy and a method for keeping the reconstituted drug cold. A generic form of epoprostenol became available in the United States in 2008, but availability has been inconsistent. Recently, a heat stable form of epoprostenol has been developed that obviates the need for ice packs in the infusion pump and allows patients to run their pump longer without refilling their reservoir.

Treprostinil is a prostacyclin analogue that is chemically altered to achieve longer half-life and also has greater stability at room air temperature. This drug was developed for subcutaneous infusion and approved for this indication in 2002. Further studies led to the FDA adding treprostinil infusion via an indwelling central venous catheter to the labeling in late 2004. Following additional development and clinical studies, treprostinil was approved for inhalational therapy in 2009 and oral therapy in 2013.

TABLE 6.1 — Prostanoid Therapies Used for the Treatment of PAH

Compound	Commercial Product	Route of Administration	Stability	Delivery Device
Epoprostenol	Flolan	Intravenous	Stable at 4°C	CADD Legacy
	Generic	Intravenous	Stable at 4°C	CADD Legacy
	Veltri	Intravenous	Stable at room air	CADD Legacy
Treprostinil	Remodulin	Intravenous infusion	Stable at room air	CADD Legacy or Cane Crono 5
	Remodulin	Subcutaneous infusion	Stable at room air	CADD-MS 3 or MiniMed 407C
	Tyvaso	Inhalation	Stable at room air	OPTINEB-ir
	Orenitram	Oral	Stable at room air	—
Iloprost	Ventavis	Inhalation	Stable at 4°C	Prodose or I-neb ADD System

Iloprost is a prostacyclin analogue initially used as an intravenous infusion to treat PAH in Europe. Further studies demonstrated that it could also be used to treat PAH when given by inhalation. Iloprost was approved for the treatment of PAH in the United States via the inhalation route in 2004, but has not been approved in the United States for intravenous infusion. In addition to the prostacyclin analogues mentioned above, a nonprostanoid, prostacyclin receptor agonist named selexipeg has been developed and recently completed clinical trials.

It is unclear if inhaled or orally active prostacyclins or prostacyclin receptor agonists are as efficacious for the treatment of PAH as parenteral prostacyclin therapy. Continuous infusion maintains circulating drug levels at a higher level than would be achieved by oral or inhalational administration. Due to a high degree of tachyphylaxis, parenteral prostacyclins are usually increased to the highest tolerable dose, often resulting in doses that are many-fold higher than what the patient is started on initially. Also, the severe side effects that are associated with even intermittent interruption of therapy result in an extremely high compliance rate among patients utilizing this form of therapy. Thus, it is difficult to compare intravenous prostanoid therapy with inhaled or oral prostacyclins.

What is clear is that some patients treated with parenteral prostacyclins have had marked improvement in their symptoms and functional capacity, and the widely held consensus among experts in the field is that the continuous infusion of intravenous epoprostenol is the most efficacious therapy that is presently available for the treatment of PAH. This opinion is reflected by professional treatment guidelines that recommend epoprostenol infusion as initial therapy in patients who present in the most advanced stages of PAH.[12,13]

It is also possible that individual variability in expression and/or activity of prostacyclin binding receptors may make one prostacyclin analogue better suited for some patients than for others. Further studies are needed to determine the extent of individual variability in prostacyclin receptor expression and if long-term prostacyclin therapy results in changes in prostacyclin receptor expression. Until these studies are completed, the different prostacyclin analogues should not be considered clinically equivalent drugs. Although inhaled and orally active prostanoids may allow patients easier access to prostacyclin therapy, failure to respond satisfactorily to inhaled or oral prostacyclins should not prevent patients from being given a trial of intravenous prostacyclin therapy. Furthermore, patients with advanced disease, particularly those who progress to WHO functional class IV, should not be given oral or inhaled prostacyclin therapy in lieu of intravenous prostacyclin therapy.[12,13]

Intravenous Prostacyclin Therapy

Randomized controlled trials of intravenous epo-prostenol and treprostinil have demonstrated both drugs to be effective in the treatment of PAH. Epoprostenol was the first of the currently approved PAH-specific therapies to be studied in a large randomized clinical trial.[1] In that landmark study, 81 patients with PAH in functional class III or IV were randomized in unblinded fashion to receive continuous intravenous infusion of epoprostenol with or without conventional therapy which included anticoagulants, oral vasodilators, diuretic agents, cardiac glycosides, and supplemental oxygen. The primary objective was to assess the effect of epoprostenol on exercise capacity in these patients with advanced PAH.

Approximately 25% of patients were in NYHA class IV at the time of study entry. At the end of the 12-week study, patients treated with epoprostenol had a mean increase in 6MWD of 32 m, whereas those treated with conventional therapy alone had a decrease of 15 m ($P<0.003$). The PVR decreased 21% in the epoprostenol group and increased 9% in the conventional therapy group ($P<0.001$). Eight patients died during the 12 weeks of study in the conventional therapy group and none in the group that received epoprostenol ($P<0.003$) (**Figure 6.1**). Although this was an unblinded study, it remains one of the only studies able to demonstrate a survival benefit. Significant improvements in 6MWD and pulmonary hemodynamics were also seen with epoprostenol infusion after 12 weeks of study in 118 patients with PAH associated with scleroderma.[14]

Intravenous treprostinil was studied in a small but placebo-controlled and double-blinded randomized trial.[15] After 12 weeks of study, the median placebo-

FIGURE 6.1 — Survival Among 41 Patients Treated With Epoprostenol and 40 Patients Receiving Conventional Therapy

6

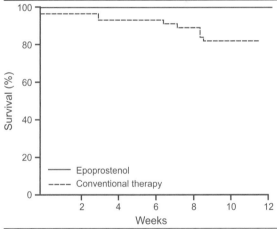

Data on patients who underwent transplantation during the 12-week study were censored at the time of transplantation. Estimates were made by the Kaplan–Meier product-limit method. The two-sided P value from the log-rank test was 0.003. Survival analysis with data on patients receiving transplants not censored at transplantation resulted in the same level of significance (two-sided $P = 0.003$ by the log-rank test).

Barst RJ, et al. *N Engl J Med*. 1996;334(5):296-301.

adjusted increase in 6MWD was 83 m ($P<0.008$). There was also a strong trend toward increased survival that did not quite reach statistical significance ($P=0.051$). No study has compared intravenous epoprostenol with intravenous treprostinil, but one study examined the effect of switching patients who were stable on intravenous epoprostenol to intravenous treprostinil.[16] In that study, 31 patients were transitioned to intravenous treprostinil over 24 to 48 hours and followed for 12 weeks. During the study period, four patients switched back to intravenous epoprostenol: three due to leg pain and one due to worsening PAH symptoms in the setting of pneumonia. In the 27 patients who remained on intravenous treprostinil, there was no change from baseline in 6MWD, Borg dyspnea score, or functional class. However, PVR index (PVRI) increased about 23% ($3+1$ mm Hg/L/m^2).

Epoprostenol is available as a lyophilized powder and reconstituted in normal saline or specially designed diluent. Treprostinil comes premixed in 20-mL vials in concentrations of 1.0, 2.5, 5.0, or 10 mg/mL. Epoprostenol is stable for 24 hours if kept on ice, and the pump reservoir must be replaced with fresh drug every day. Heat stable epoprostenol and treprostinil remain stable at room temperature for 72 hours, and patients can go 3 days before replacing the reservoir with freshly prepared drug.

Infusion is delivered by programmable battery-operated pumps equipped with alarms that indicate interruption of drug delivery and alert the patient to when their reservoir is nearing empty (**Figure 6.2**). Drug dose is determined by the concentration and infusion rate. Therapy is usually initiated at 1-2 ng/kg/min and the dose increased in increments of 0.5-1 ng/kg/min every 30 to 60 minutes until signs of systemic effects are seen. Systemic effects include facial flushing, headache, jaw pain, nausea, diarrhea, and pain in the long bones of the legs or bottom of the feet. The goal of prostacyclin therapy is to administer the maximum dose that is comfortable for the patient.

FIGURE 6.2 — Portable Infusion Pumps Used to Administer Intravenous Epoprostenol, Treprostinil, or Subcutaneous Treprostinil

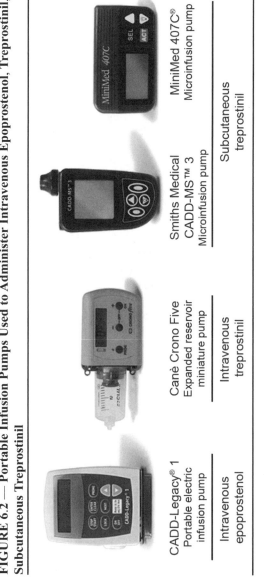

CADD-Legacy® 1
Portable electric
infusion pump

Intravenous
epoprostenol

Canè Crono Five
Expanded reservoir
miniature pump

Intravenous
treprostinil

Smiths Medical
CADD-MS™ 3
Microinfusion pump

MiniMed 407C®
Microinfusion pump

Subcutaneous
treprostinil

Patients need not suffer the adverse effects of prostacyclin infusion to fully reap its benefits, but it is reassuring to both patient and physician when a little flushing or jaw pain is present to ensure that there is enough drug on board to cause some systemic effects. Due to a high level of tachyphylaxis, the dose is usually increased daily or every other day for the first week or two. By the end of the first month, patients can often go for 1 to 2 weeks before increasing their infusion rate. After several months of therapy, patients are usually able to stay on a steady dose of drug, but they should continue to attempt a small dose increase about once each month to make sure they are near the highest tolerable dose.

Intravenous prostanoid therapies require a secure central venous access such as a Hickman catheter for their administration. Once prostacyclin infusion therapy has been initiated, patients quickly become dependent on its pulmonary vasodilator effects. Even a brief interruption can result in rebound pulmonary hypertension and hemodynamic instability, especially if they are not on any other PAH-specific medication. Extravasation of prostacyclin that has been adminis-tered via peripheral IV access can also cause significant edema and local skin irritation (**Figure 6.3**). If central venous access is lost in the course of infusion therapy, prostacyclin can be administered via a peripheral IV, but central venous access should be re-established as quickly as possible to ensure secure access.

Not all patients are appropriate candidates for prostacyclin infusion therapy. Patients must be able to mix drug, keep their central catheter clean and func-tioning, operate and troubleshoot their infusion pump, and maintain sterile technique while changing the tubing that connects to their central line. Patients must also be able to obtain medical care quickly in the event of a central line infection or failure. Preferably, patients should have a partner who is with them most of the time and is able to operate their pump in the event that the patient becomes ill or incapacitated. Patients must

FIGURE 6.3 — Local Erythema and Edema Caused by Extravasation of Epoprostenol Following Administration Through Peripheral IV

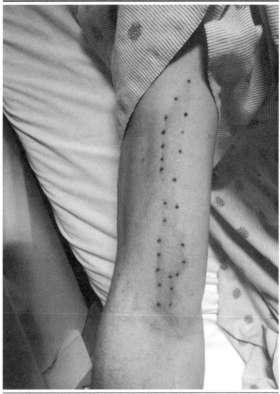

The patient's central line catheter had become dislodged and epoprostenol was administered via a standard IV placed in the antecubital fossa while new central access was being obtained. The skin lesions resolved within 24 hours of discontinuing the peripheral IV.

understand that they are the first line of expertise for their medical therapy. Most medical facilities, rescue personnel, and even emergency room physicians will not be familiar with prostacyclin therapy and are unable to troubleshoot their infusion pump. Intravenous infusion therapy is usually delivered by centers with expertise and experience in this type of care that can provide a 24-hour emergency contact if the patient experiences acute problems.

Central line infection and dysfunction are a common consequence of prostacyclin infusion therapy. Approximately 10% of patients on this therapy will experience central line infection and/or bacteremia per each year of use. Outbreaks of staph micrococcus have been reported with epoprostenol, and Gram-negative bacteremia appears to be more frequent in patients treated with intravenous treprostinil infusion.[17] Guidelines for the prevention of catheter-related, blood-stream infections have been published by the Scientific Leadership Council of the Pulmonary Hypertension Association.[18] In addition to infection, central catheters also develop leaks, breaks, or dislodgement and usually have to be replaced every 2 to 3 years.

Subcutaneous Prostacyclin Infusion

Treprostinil is the only prostacyclin approved for subcutaneous administration and must be given as a continuous subcutaneous infusion. It is generally infused at doses similar or slightly higher than those used with intravenous epoprostenol infusion and with the same need for frequent adjustments to achieve the maximal dose that is comfortable for the patient. Subcutaneous infusion has several advantages over intravenous infusion. The most obvious is the lack of need for a central catheter. The other is that subcutaneous infusion rates are much lower, on the order of hundredths of a mL/hr and a 3-mL reservoir generally holds enough drug to last for 3 days of continuous infusion. As a result, the portable infusion pump is considerably smaller (**Figure 6.2**). Subcutaneous infusion also provides a longer period before drug is depleted if the infusion is interrupted. Patients usually have a window of several hours after infusion is stopped before becoming symptomatic. Subcutaneous therapy may be easier for some patients to manage, particularly those who have difficulty mixing drug, caring for a central venous catheter, or who do not have rapid access to a health care facility in the event of drug interruption.

It is unclear if subcutaneous infusion is as effective as intravenous prostanoid infusion. Concerns have been raised that less drug is absorbed from subcutaneous tissues than is delivered by direct IV infusion. Infusion site discomfort may also prevent patients from increasing their dose, even though a higher dose is not usually associated with more intense site pain. In the only large randomized placebo-controlled trial of subcutaneous infusion of treprostinil for treatment of PAH, improvement in 6MWD capacity correlated with the dose of drug achieved at study end.[19] In that study, 470 patients with idiopathic PAH or PAH associated with scleroderma or congenital heart disease were randomized to receive subcutaneous infusion of treprostinil or placebo. The primary outcome variable was the placebo corrected change in 6MWD test which was only 16 m greater in the treprostinil-treated group than in the placebo group. However, the improvement in 6MWD was greater in patients who were in the highest quartile of treprostinil dose at the end of the study (**Figure 6.4**). For patients who had a dose of >13.8 ng/kg/min, the placebo adjusted increase in 6MWD was 33 m, similar to that achieved in other studies of prostacyclin infusion.[1,14]

The primary disadvantage of subcutaneous infusion is the discomfort that occurs at the skin infusion site. Infusion sites are usually placed in areas rich in adipose tissue, such as the lower quadrants of the abdomen or in the fatty aspects of the upper arms or buttocks. The severity of discomfort varies considerably between patients and between infusion sites in the same patient. A variety of topical ointments or pain relievers have been used to help patients tolerate the discomfort, but in the study mentioned above,[19] 8% of

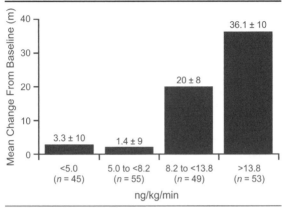

Simonneau G, et al. *Am J Respir Crit Care Med.* 2002;165(6):800-804.

patients had to discontinue subcutaneous infusion due to inability to control infusion site pain. In general, site pain is worse during the initial few days of infusion. Once comfortable, patients can utilize the same infusion site for many weeks at a time. If pain control cannot be accomplished, switching to a new infusion site is recommended.

Adverse effects are similar to those of intravenous infusion. Skin site infections including cellulitis and abscess formation are uncommon and can be difficult to distinguish from the mild skin swelling, warmth, and erythema produced by treprostinil. Signs of abscess formation or infection include increasing tenderness, fluctuance, and purulent drainage from the site. If caught early, changing the infusion site may alleviate the problem, but if an abscess develops, incision and drainage of the site and antibiotic therapy may be needed.

Treprostinil and iloprost have both been approved as inhalation therapy to treat PAH in the United States. Each is delivered by a specially designed nebulizer-delivery device that can only be used with the drug it was designed for. Both inhaled drugs reach peak plasma levels within minutes of inhalation and are rapidly cleared from the circulation following completion of the treatment. The plasma clearance half-lives for iloprost and treprostinil upon completion of the approved inhaled dose are approximately 8 and 45 minutes, respectively (**Figure 6.5**). Thus, inhaled therapy with either drug produces substantial periods between treatments when no drug can be detected in the circulation. The complete clearance of drug between treatments means that a steady state drug level is never achieved.

Although it is possible that some drug remains active within the lung, it is unlikely that there is any significant vasodilator effect that is active by the time the next dose is taken. The loss of vasodilator effect has been well demonstrated with inhaled iloprost. In the seminal study that led to its approval in the United States,[20] mPAP and PVR decreased and cardiac output improved following a single dose of inhaled iloprost. After 12 weeks of treatment that consisted of six to nine inhalations a day, mPAP, PVR, and cardiac output were all significantly improved from baseline if measured after completion of therapy but were unchanged from baseline if measured prior to treatment (**Table 6.2**). The intermittent effect of inhaled prostacyclin therapy has caused speculation as to whether it is as effective as continuous infusion therapy.

In the above study,[20] patients treated with inhaled iloprost alone were more likely to achieve a composite endpoint of a 10% or greater improvement in 6MWD and improvement of at least one NYHA functional class in the absence of clinical deterioration or death

FIGURE 6.5 — Plasma Levels Plotted Against Time of Iloprost and Treprostinil During and After a Single Inhalation Treatment

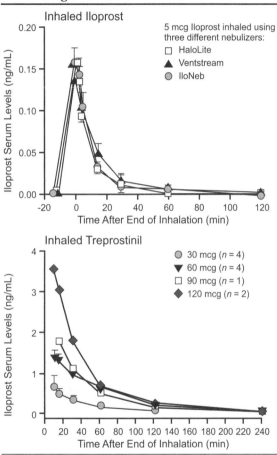

For iloprost, peak blood levels are achieved within 5 minutes of inhalation and the T½ is 6.5-9.4 minutes. For treprostinil, peak plasma levels occur within 10-15 minutes of inhalation and the T½ is 44-52 minutes.

Olschewski H, et al. *Chest*. 2003;124(4):1294-1304. Channick RN, et al. *J Am Coll Cardiol*. 2006;48(7):1433-1437.

TABLE 6.2 — Change From Baseline Hemodynamic Measurements After 12 Weeks of Inhaled Placebo or Iloprost

	Placebo Group	Iloprost Group	
		Before Inhalation	After Inhalation
Pulmonary-artery pressure (mm Hg)	-0.2 ± 6.9	-0.1 ± 7.3	-4.6 ± 9.3[a]
Cardiac output (liters/min)	-0.19 ± 0.81[b]	$+0.05 \pm 0.86$	$+0.55 \pm 1.1$[a]
Pulmonary vascular resistance (dyn·sec·cm^{-5})	$+96 \pm 322$[b]	-9 ± 275[c]	-239 ± 279[a]

N = 146 patients.

[a] $P < 0.001$ for the difference from baseline values.
[b] $P < 0.05$ for the difference from baseline values.
[c] $P < 0.01$ for the comparison with the placebo group.

Olschewski H, et al: Aerosolized Iloprost Randomized Study Group. *N Engl J Med.* 2002;347(5):322-329.

than controls. The efficacy of long-term iloprost inhalation therapy has not been well studied, but in one report, nearly a third of patients (19/63) examined discontinued therapy and the 2-year calculated survival rate was 87% compared with a 63% predicted survival rate.[21] Several studies have also demonstrated improvement in functional capacity when inhaled iloprost is added to a background therapy of PDE5I or endothelin receptor antagonist (ERA).[22,23]

The short half-life of inhaled iloprost requires between six to nine treatments per day to be effective, and some patients may require treatments in the middle of the night as well. Syncope and other adverse events have been reported between treatments and attributed to the fall in plasma drug levels, although the incidence of these events has been very low.[20,21] Iloprost is delivered via a portable, battery-operated nebulizer device (**Figure 6.6**). Each treatment takes between 5 to 10 minutes to complete, depending on the rate and depth of breathing.

Inhaled treprostinil was developed with the idea that its longer half-life would allow for less frequent treatments. The stability of treprostinil at room temperature allows for the portable nebulizer (**Figure 6.6**) to be loaded with drug once daily, and the delivery device was designed to complete a treatment with only three to nine breaths. These alterations have resulted in an inhaled prostanoid treatment that is more convenient for patients to use. However, inhaled treprostinil has not been studied as monotherapy for PAH. In the only large clinical trial that has been conducted (TRIUMPH), inhaled treprostinil or placebo given 4 times daily was randomly assigned to patients with PAH who were on background therapy with either sildenafil or bosentan.[24] Compared with placebo, patients assigned to inhaled treprostinil had a significant improvement in 6MWD, the primary endpoint of the study, after 3 months of treatment. The results of this study led to the approval of inhaled treprostinil for functional class II or III patients who are already being

FIGURE 6.6 — Portable Nebulizers Designed for Use With Inhaled Iloprost or Treprostinil

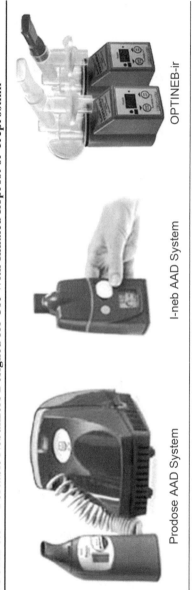

Prodose AAD System

I-neb AAD System

OPTINEB-ir

The Prodose and I-neb Adaptive Aerosol Delivery (AAD) System are used for delivery of inhaled iloprost and the OPTINEB-ir is used for delivery of inhaled treprostinil.

treated with a PDE5 inhibitor or ERA. It is presently unknown if inhaled treprostinil alone is effective for the treatment of PAH.

Oral Prostacyclins

Two orally active agents have been studied for the treatment of PAH. Oral treprostinil was approved for the treatment of PAH at the end of 2014. The drug is made orally active via a specially designed capsule that allows the slow sustained release of treprostinil via small pores drilled into its membrane. Patients are usually started at a dose of 0.25 mg twice daily and the dose is increased at regular intervals to achieve a maximum tolerable dose.

A series of clinical trials, referred to as the Freedom studies, demonstrated moderate efficacy. The first large randomized controlled study examined the efficacy of oral treprostinil vs placebo in treatment-naïve patients with PAH.[25] A modified intention-to-treat cohort that included 228 patients (151 received treprostinil, 77 received placebo) who had access to a lower dose (0.25-mg) tablet that allowed for better dose adjustment was studied. In this group of patients, there was a treatment effect for 6MWD of 23.0 m ($P=0.0125$) after 12 weeks of study. No change in secondary endpoints that included Borg dyspnea index, clinical worsening, and symptoms of PAH was observed. The most common adverse events were headache (69%), nausea (39%), diarrhea (37%), and jaw pain.

Two additional clinical trials have examined the efficacy of oral treprostinil when added to a background therapy of a PDE5 inhibitor and/or ERA. In the first study,[26] 350 patients were randomized to oral treprostinil or placebo. 63 patients did not complete the 16-week study. In the remainder, there was an 11 m improvement in 6MWD that did not quite reach statistical significance ($P=0.07$), but there were improvements in a dyspnea-fatigue index score. It was also noted that improvement in the 6MWD correlated with the dose of drug used. Patients who had achieved a dose of 1-3.25 mg/day by end of study had an 18 m improvement in 6MWD and those who had achieved a dose of 3.5-16 mg/day had an improvement of 34 m. In a follow-up study,[27] dosing was modified to achieve higher drug levels and the mean dose at end of study was $3.1 + 1.9$ mg/day. In this study,[27] 310 patients with PAH already receiving a stable dose of PDE5 inhibitor and/or ERA were randomized 1:1 to receive oral treprostinil or placebo. Despite the higher dose achieved, the change in 6MWD was only 10 m and was not significantly different from controls ($P=0.89$). No changes in secondary endpoints including WHO functional class, Borg dyspnea score, dyspnea-fatigue index, signs and symptoms of PAH, or clinical worsening were seen.

Recently published treatment guidelines for PAH were developed just prior to the time of FDA approval for oral treprostinil. As a result, there has been little opportunity for professional societies and clinical experts to determine how oral treprostinil should best be used. Most experts agree that it is reasonable to add oral treprostinil to background treatment with a PDE5 inhibitor or ERA in functional class II or III patients with Group 1 PAH who have failed to reach their treatment goals. It may also be reasonable to consider oral treprostinil for treatment-naïve patients who are unable to tolerate a PDE5 inhibitor or ERA. However, oral treprostinil should not be used in place of parenteral prostacyclin therapy in patients who present in functional class IV or in functional class III patients who are deteriorating.

Beraprost is another orally active prostacyclin derivative. Data supporting its efficacy in PAH are limited. Initial studies suggested favorable effects that ultimately led to its approval for the treatment of PAH in Japan,[28,29] but additional studies suggested that its beneficial effects were not sustained during longer-term treatment.[30] Beraprost is not approved for the treatment of PAH in the United States but is presently undergoing study as an add-on agent to inhaled treprostinil. The completion of these studies will be necessary before determining if this is a successful method of treating PAH.

Summary

Prostacyclin remains one of the most important options in the treatment of PAH. When given as a continuous intravenous infusion with regular dose escalation to maintain maximally tolerated levels, it may be the most efficacious treatment available for PAH. The development of different prostacyclin analogues such as treprostinil and iloprost has resulted in the ability to administer prostacyclins by subcutaneous infusion, inhalation, and by orally active tablet. These newer approaches have made prostacyclin therapy more manageable and likely have provided greater access to this class of drug than was previously available.

However, it is not known if all prostacyclin analogs are as effective as intravenous epoprostenol, and they should not be used interchangeably. Present guidelines for the treatment of PAH recommend the use of subcutaneous, inhaled, or orally active prostacyclin analogues for patients in functional class II or III, but clearly stipulate that patients who progress to functional class IV or who present in functional class IV should be treated with intravenous epoprostenol.

Key Points

- Currently available prostanoids therapies for the treatment of PAH can be administered as continuous intravenous or subcutaneous infusion, frequent inhalation, or twice daily oral ingestion.
- The comparative efficacy of parenteral, inhaled, and oral prostanoids has not been studied, but

currently available prostacyclin-derived medications are unlikely to be equivalent.

- Intravenous epoprostenol is generally considered to be the most efficacious treatment for PAH and should be highly considered for use in patients who present in or deteriorate to NYHA functional class IV.
- The expanding number of prostanoids treatment options allows better access for PAH patients to this group of medications but should not impede patients with advanced disease from receiving intravenous infusion therapy.

6

REFERENCES

1. Barst RJ, Rubin LJ, Long WA, et al; Primary Pulmonary Hypertension Study Group. A comparison of continuous intravenous epoprostenol (prostacyclin) with conventional therapy for primary pulmonary hypertension. *N Engl J Med.* 1996;334(5):296-301.

2. Moncada S, Gryglewski R, Bunting S, Vane JR. An enzyme isolated from arteries transforms prostaglandin endoperoxides to an unstable substance that inhibits platelet aggregation. *Nature.* 1976;263(5579):663-665.

3. Whittaker N, Bunting S, Salmon J, et al. The chemical structure of prostaglandin X (prostacyclin). *Prostaglandins.* 1976;12(6):915-928.

4. Moncada S, Higgs EA, Vane JR. Human arterial and venous tissues generate prostacyclin (prostaglandin x), a potent inhibitor of platelet aggregation. *Lancet.* 1977;1(8001):18-20.

5. Weksler BB, Marcus AJ, Jaffe EA. Synthesis of prostaglandin I2 (prostacyclin) by cultured human and bovine endothelial cells. *Proc Natl Acad Sci USA.* 1977;74(9):3922-3926.

6. Gryglewski RJ. Prostaglandins, platelets, and atherosclerosis. *CRC Crit Rev Biochem.* 1980;7(4):291-338. Review.

7. Hyman AL, Chapnick BM, Kadowitz PJ, et al. Unusual pulmonary vasodilator activity of 13,14-dehydroprostacyclin methyl ester: comparison with endoperoxides and other prostanoids. *Proc Natl Acad Sci USA.* 1977;74(12):5711-5715.

8. Christman BW, McPherson CD, Newman JH, et al. An imbalance between the excretion of thromboxane and prostacyclin metabolites in pulmonary hypertension. *N Engl J Med.* 1992;327:70-75.

9. Tuder RM, Cool CD, Geraci MW, et al. Prostacyclin synthase expression is decreased in lungs from patients with severe pulmonary hypertension. *Am J Respir Crit Care Med.* 1999;159:1925-1932.

10. Gorman RR, Bunting S, Miller OV. Modulation of human platelet adenylate cyclase by prostacyclin (PGX). *Prostaglandins.* 1977;13(3):377-388.

11. Falcetti E, Flavell DM, Staels B, Tinker A, Haworth SG, Clapp LH. IP receptor-dependent activation of PPARgamma by stable prostacyclin analogues. *Biochem Biophys Res Commun.* 2007;360(4):821-827.

12. Taichman DB, Ornelas J, Chung L, et al. Pharmacologic therapy for pulmonary arterial hypertension in adults: CHEST guideline and expert panel report. *Chest*. 2014;146(2):449-475.

13. Galiè N, Corris PA, Frost A, et al. Updated treatment algorithm of pulmonary arterial hypertension. *J Am Coll Cardiol*. 2013;62(25 suppl):D60-D72.

14. Badesch DB, Tapson VF, McGoon MD, et al. Continuous intravenous epoprostenol for pulmonary hypertension due to the scleroderma spectrum of disease. A randomized, controlled trial. *Ann Intern Med*. 2000;132(6):425-434.

15. Hiremath J, Thanikachalam S, Parikh K, et al; TRUST Study Group. Exercise improvement and plasma biomarker changes with intravenous treprostinil therapy for pulmonary arterial hypertension: a placebo-controlled trial. *J Heart Lung Transplant*. 2010;29(2):137-149.

16. Gomberg-Maitland M, Tapson VF, Benza RL, et al. Transition from intravenous epoprostenol to intravenous treprostinil in pulmonary hypertension. *Am J Respir Crit Care Med*. 2005;172(12):1586-1589.

17. Centers for Disease Control and Prevention (CDC). Bloodstream infections among patients treated with intravenous epoprostenol or intravenous treprostinil for pulmonary arterial hypertension--seven sites, United States, 2003-2006. *MMWR Morb Mortal Wkly Rep*. 2007;56(8):170-172.

18. Doran AK, Ivy DD, Barst RJ, Hill N, Murali S, Benza RL; Scientific Leadership Council of the Pulmonary Hypertension Association. Guidelines for the prevention of central venous catheter-related blood stream infections with prostanoids therapy for pulmonary arterial hypertension. *Int J Clin Pract Suppl*. 2008;(160):5-9.

19. Simonneau G, Barst RJ, Galie N, et al; Treprostinil Study Group. Continuous subcutaneous infusion of treprostinil, a prostacyclin analogue, in patients with pulmonary arterial hypertension: a double-blind, randomized, placebo-controlled trial. *Am J Respir Crit Care Med*. 2002;165(6):800-804.

20. Olschewski H, Simonneau G, Galiè N, et al; Aerosolized Iloprost Randomized Study Group. Inhaled iloprost for severe pulmonary hypertension. *N Engl J Med*. 2002;347(5):322-329.

21. Olschewski H, Hoeper MM, Behr J, et al. Long-term therapy with inhaled iloprost in patients with pulmonary hypertension. *Respir Med*. 2010;104(5):731-740.

6

22. Ghofrani HA, Wiedemann R, Rose F, et al. Combination therapy with oral sildenafil and inhaled iloprost for severe pulmonary hypertension. *Ann Intern Med*. 2002;136:515-522.

23. McLaughlin VV, Oudiz RJ, Frost A, et al. Randomized study of adding inhaled iloprost to existing bosentan in pulmonary arterial hypertension. *Am J Respir Crit Care Med*. 2006;174:1257-1263.

24. McLaughlin VV, Benza RL, Rubin LJ, et al. Addition of inhaled treprostinil to oral therapy for pulmonary arterial hypertension: a randomized controlled clinical trial. *J Am Coll Cardiol*. 2010;55:1915-1922.

25. Jing ZC, Parikh K, Pulido T, et al. Efficacy and safety of oral treprostinil monotherapy for the treatment of pulmonary arterial hypertension: a randomized, controlled trial. *Circulation*. 2013;127(5):624-633.

26. Tapson VF, Torres F, Kermeen F, et al. Oral treprostinil for the treatment of pulmonary arterial hypertension in patients on background endothelin receptor antagonist and/or phosphodiesterase type 5 inhibitor therapy (the FREEDOM-C study): a randomized controlled trial. *Chest*. 2012;142(6):1383-1390.

27. Tapson VF, Jing ZC, Xu KF, et al; FREEDOM-C2 Study Team. Oral treprostinil for the treatment of pulmonary arterial hypertension in patients receiving background endothelin receptor antagonist and phosphodiesterase type 5 inhibitor therapy (the FREEDOM-C2 study): a randomized controlled trial. *Chest*. 2013;144(3):952-958.

28. Nagaya N, Uematsu M, Okano Y, et al. Effect of orally active prostacyclin analogue on survival of outpatients with primary pulmonary hypertension. *J Am Coll Cardiol*. 1999;34(4):1188-1192.

29. Galiè N, Humbert M, Vachiéry JL, et al; Arterial Pulmonary Hypertension and Beraprost European (ALPHABET) Study Group. Effects of beraprost sodium, an oral prostacyclin analogue, in patients with pulmonary arterial hypertension: a randomized, double-blind, placebo-controlled trial. *J Am Coll Cardiol*. 2002;39(9):1496-1502.

30. Barst RJ, McGoon M, McLaughlin V, et al; Beraprost Study Group. Beraprost therapy for pulmonary arterial hypertension. *J Am Coll Cardiol*. 2003;41(12):2119-2125.

7 Endothelin Receptor Antagonists

*by Arunabh Talwar, MD and
Sonu Sahni, MD*

Endothelins (ET) are 21-amino acid peptides implicated in vasoconstriction which are primarily produced in the endothelium and play a major role in vascular hemodynamics. Endothelins are also the culprit in vascular diseases of several organ systems, including the heart, general circulation, and the pulmonary vascular system.[1] Vascular endothelial cells are the major source of endothelin-1 (ET-1) production in humans and play an important role in controlling vascular smooth vessel tone. ET-1 is mainly secreted abluminally toward vascular smooth muscle cells, suggesting a paracrine role.[2] ET-1 expression is increased in pulmonary vascular endothelial cells in patients with PAH, and plasma ET-1 levels correlate directly with PAP and mortality. In contrast, ET-1 receptor antagonists (ERA) have been shown to blunt the development of PH in animals and to reduce PAP and delay time to clinical worsening in patients with PAH. Several ERAs have been developed and are approved for the treatment of patients with WHO Group 1 PAH.

Mechanism of Action

The two distinct receptors for endothelin are connected to guanine nucleotide-binding (G) proteins. ET-A receptors are primarily expressed on pulmonary vascular smooth muscle cells, whereas ET-B receptors are located on both pulmonary vascular endothelial cells and smooth muscle cells. When activated, the ET-A receptor mediates vasoconstriction via G protein-induced phospholipase C activation, 1,4,5-inositol triphosphate (IP3) formation, and the consequent release of Ca^{2+} from intracellular stores.[3] Increased IP3 causes calcium release by the sarcoplasmic reticulum which causes smooth muscle contraction.[4] Other effects of ET-1 on pulmonary vascular cells are illustrated in **Figure 7.1**.[5]

In addition to mediating vasoconstriction, ET-1 is also a potent mitogen and has been implemented in cellular proliferation of many cell types, including vascular smooth muscle cells[6] which contribute to reduced compliance of the pulmonary vasculature and leads to increased PVR.

ET-B receptors on endothelial cells mediate vasodilation via increased production of nitric oxide and prostacyclins. In addition to potentially mediating pulmonary vasodilation, the ET-B receptor may also mediate a vasoconstrictive effect through a population of ET-B receptors located on vascular smooth muscle cells.[7]

ERAs and PAH

In patients with idiopathic and secondary PH, the ET-1 expression in pulmonary tissue is increased.[4] The synthesis of endothelin is regulated by a variety of factors such as pulsatile stretch, acidosis, and hypoxia.[8-10] Hypoxia, in particular, is a strong stimulus for ET-1 synthesis.[10] Furthermore, vasoconstrictors,[11] growth factors,[12] and adhesion molecules[13] also stimulate ET production. Inhibitors of ET-1 synthesis include NO,[14] prostacyclin,[15] and some estrogens.[16]

ET receptor antagonism is frequently used as an initial therapy for PAH. Both ET-A and ET-B receptors are expressed on the surface of smooth muscle cells where vasoconstriction and cellular proliferation take place and where ET receptor antagonists are active. Both nonselective and ET-A selective agents have been developed for the treatment of PAH (**Table 7.1**). Bosentan, the first ERA developed for PAH, antagonizes both ET-A and ET-B. Ambrisentan and macitentan have much greater selectivity for ET-A.

154

FIGURE 7.1 — Endothelin (ET)-1 in PAH

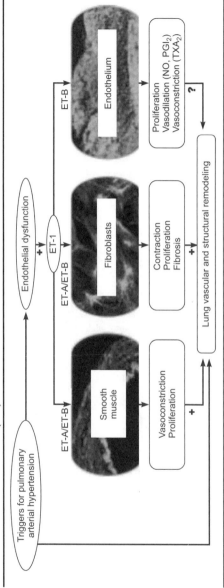

Key: + = stimulation; ? = unknown effect.

Adapted from Dupuis J, et al. *Eur Respir J.* 2008;31(2):407-415.

TABLE 7.1 — Endothelin Receptor Antagonist Pharmacokinetic Characteristics

Characteristics	Ambrisentan	Bosentan	Macitentan
Half-life/dosing interval	15 hours/once daily	5 hours/twice daily	16 hours/once daily
Receptor binding	Endothelin receptor-A	Endothelin receptor-A/ Endothelin receptor-B	Endothelin receptor-A/ Endothelin receptor-B
Bioavailability	Unknown, unaffected by food	50%, unaffected by food	Unknown, unaffected by food
Metabolism	Hepatic phase 2 glucuronidation	Hepatic CYP450	Hepatic CYP 450 3A4 and 2C19
Excretion	Biliary	Biliary	Renal, fecal
CYP interactions	Minimal with CYP2C9, CYP3A4, or CYP1A2	Induces CYP2C9, CYP3A4; possibly CYP2C19	No induction or inhibition of CYP enzymes

Letairis [package insert]. Foster City, CA: Gilead Sciences, Inc; October 2015; Tracleer [package insert]. South San Francisco, CA: Actelion Pharmaceuticals US, Inc; October 2015; Opsumit [package insert]. South San Francisco, CA: Actelion Pharmaceuticals US, Inc; April 2015; Barst RJ. *Vasc Health Risk Manag*. 2007;3:11-22; Wrisheo RE. *J Clin Pharmacol*. 2008;48:610-618.

Bosentan

The dual ET-1 receptor blocker bosentan is an orally active nonpeptide ERA that was shown to reduce PAP, pulmonary vascular remodeling, and right ventricular hypertrophy, without inducing systemic vasodilatation in a rat model of chronic pulmonary hypertension.[17] Acute administration of high doses of bosentan in PAH patients produced a decrease in PVR and systemic vascular resistance (SVR) which suggested that chronic doses may provide clinically significant effect.[18] Bosentan received FDA approval in November 2001 for patients with WHO Group 1 PAH in functional class III or IV. A more recent study also found clinical efficacy in PAH patients in functional class II.

Initial studies by Channick and colleagues randomized 32 patients with PAH, functional class III, to bosentan or placebo for 12 weeks. In the bosentan group, the 6MWD improved by 70 m at 12 weeks compared with baseline, whereas it worsened by 6 m in those on placebo (difference 76 m [95% CI 12-139], $P=0.021$). The improvement was maintained for at least 20 weeks. The cardiac index was 1.0 L/min–1 m–2 (95% CI 0.6-1.4; $P<0.0001$) greater in patients given bosentan than in those given placebo. PVR decreased by 223 dyn·sec·cm^{-5} with bosentan, but increased by 191 dyn·sec·cm^{-5} with placebo (difference -415 [-608 to -221]; $P=0.0002$). Patients given bosentan had a reduced Borg dyspnea index and an improved WHO functional class. All three withdrawals due to clinical worsening were in the placebo group ($P=0.033$). The number and nature of adverse events did not differ between the two groups (**Figure 7.2**).[19]

Efficacy was further confirmed by the subsequent BREATHE-1 (Bosentan Randomized Trial of Endothelin Antagonist Therapy) trial.[20] This trial randomized 213 patients with idiopathic PAH (70%) or PAH associated with connective tissue disease (30%) who were NYHA functional classes III and IV

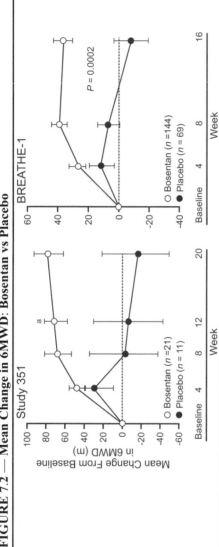

FIGURE 7.2 — Mean Change in 6MWD: Bosentan vs Placebo

[a] P <0.05 vs baseline; P = 0.021 vs placebo. Values are mean ± SEM.

Modified from Channick RN, et al. *Lancet*. 2001;358:1119-1123. Rubin LJ, et al. *N Engl J Med*. 2002;346:896-903.

to placebo or bosentan at a dosage of 125 mg or 250 mg twice daily. After 16 weeks of therapy, patients treated with bosentan had an improved 6MWD; the mean difference between the placebo group and the combined bosentan groups was 44 m (95% CI, 21 to 67; $P<0.001$). Improvement was also noted in the Borg dyspnea index and WHO functional class, and there was an increased time to clinical worsening. Increases in liver aminotransferases greater than 8 times the upper limit of normal was noted in the bosentan group and was dosage-dependent with two patients in the 125-mg group and five patients in the 250-mg group.[20]

The above studies demonstrated safety and efficacy in patients with advanced pulmonary hypertensive disease. Bosentan was also studied in NYHA functional class II patients.[21] A randomized controlled trial of bosentan in less functionally impaired patients with PAH, known as the EARLY study (Endothelin Antagonist Trial in Mildly Symptomatic Pulmonary Arterial Hypertension Patients) was conducted in 185 patients with idiopathic PAH or PAH associated with connective tissue disease, congenital heart disease, or HIV infection in WHO functional class II. After 6 months of treatment, PVR, the primary outcome measure, was 83.2% of baseline (95% CI 73.8-93.7) in the bosentan group and 107.5% of baseline in the placebo group. The treatment effect was -22% in favor of bosentan ($P<0.001$). The mean 6MWD, increased from baseline in the bosentan group (11.2 m, 95% CI -4.6-27.0) and decreased in the placebo group (-7.9 m, -24.3-8.5) with a mean treatment effect of 19.1 m (95% CI 3.6-41.8; $P=0.0758$). Although the treatment effect did not reach statistical significance, patients assigned to bosentan had significant improvements in secondary outcome measures including PAP, time to clinical worsening, WHO functional class, NT-BNP levels, and feeling better as assessed by the SF-36 health transition index. Twelve (13%) patients in the bosentan group and eight (9%) in the placebo group reported serious adverse events, the most common being syncope in the bosentan group and right ventricular failure in the placebo group.[20] The mean change in 6MWD in mildly symptomatic patients in the EARLY study is shown in **Figure 7.3**.[21]

Additionally, a randomized controlled trial in patients with congenital heart disease was conducted. The BREATHE-5 study showed that in a group of patients with either atrial or ventricular septal defects, bosentan improved 6MWD without worsening hypoxemia.[22]

Bosentan dosing and monitoring information is shown in **Table 7.2**.

Ambrisentan

Due to the vasodilatory effect of ET-B, some investigators have questioned whether selective ET-A receptor antagonists would be preferable over dual antagonism. This approach would allow blockade of most of the pulmonary vasoconstrictor effect of ET-1 but preserve its vasodilatory and antimitogenic activity through unimpeded activation of the endothelial ET-B receptor.[23] Ambrisentan is a selective ET-A receptor antagonist that is indicated for the treatment of PAH (WHO Group 1):

- To improve exercise ability and delay clinical worsening
- In combination with tadalafil, to reduce the risk of disease progression and hospitalization for worsening PAH, and to improve exercise ability.

Studies establishing effectiveness included predominantly patients with WHO functional class II-III symptoms and etiologies of IPAH or HPAH (60%) or PAH associated with connective tissue diseases (34%).

After demonstrating a favorable safety and efficacy profile in an initial dosing study,[24] two randomized controlled trials, ARIES-1 and ARIES-2 (ARIES-1, 5 or 10 mg vs placebo; ARIES-2, 2.5 or 5 mg vs placebo), were conducted.[25]

In total, there were 394 patients enrolled and both trials showed improvement in the primary endpoint

FIGURE 7.3 — Mean Change in 6MWD in Mildly Symptomatic Patients (EARLY Study)

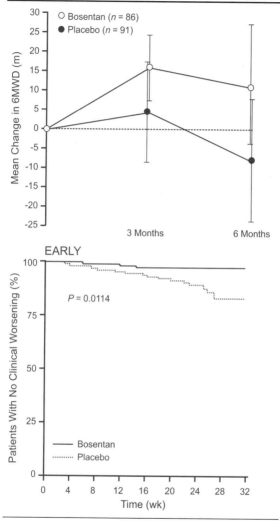

Galiè N, et al. *Lancet*. 2008;371(9630):2093-2100.

TABLE 7.2 — Bosentan Dosing and Monitoring Information

Dosing interval	Twice daily
Starting dose	62.5 mg for 4 weeks
Usual dose	125 mg
Renal impairment adjustment	None
Hepatic impairment dose adjustment	Mild: administer with caution
	Moderate to severe: avoid
LFT monitoring schedule	Liver aminotransferase levels at baseline and then monthly
When to discontinue	Aminotransferase elevations are dose-dependent. Discontinue bosentan if liver aminotransferase elevations are accompanied by clinical symptoms of hepatotoxicity (such as nausea, vomiting, fever, abdominal pain, jaundice, or unusual lethargy or fatigue) or increases of bilirubin $\geq 2 \times$ ULN
Adverse reactions	Respiratory tract infection
	Headache
	Edema
	Chest pain
	Syncope
	Flushing
	Hypotension
	Sinusitis
	Arthralgia
	Serum aminotransferases, abnormal
	Palpitations
	Anemia

Tracleer [package insert]. South San Francisco, CA: Actelion Pharmaceuticals US, Inc; October 2015.

of placebo-corrected 6MWD (**Figure 7.4** and **Figure 7.5**). In ARIES-2, there was a significant improvement in time to clinical worsening in the treatment group compared with the placebo group. There was also a trend toward improvement in time to clinical worsening in the ARIES-1 study, but it was not statistically significant. NYHA functional class improvement was significant in ARIES-1 and there was observed improvement in ARIES-2, but again it was not found to be statistically significance. A total of 298 patients were enrolled and followed in a long-term extension study (ARIES-E) over 48 weeks. Eighteen patients required additional therapies (prostanoids or phosphodiesterase type-5 [PDE5] inhibitors). Of the 280 patients continued on ambrisentan monotherapy, the improvement in 6MWD at 12 weeks was 40 m and maintained at 39 m by week 48.[25] The most commonly observed adverse

7

FIGURE 7.4 — Mean Change From Baseline in the 6MWD at Week 12 in the Placebo and Ambrisentan Groups of ARIES-1

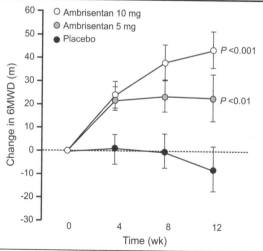

P values are vs placebo.

Galiè N, et al. *Circulation*. 2008;117:3010-3019.

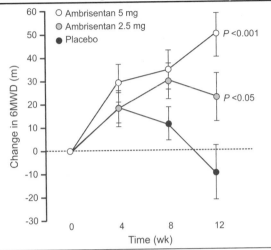

P values are vs placebo.

Galiè N, et al. *Circulation*. 2008;117:3010-3019.

events were peripheral edema, headache, and nasal congestion. No significant elevations in liver transaminase levels were observed in the ambrisentan group.

An extension study was available (ARIES-E) for patients that were included in the ARIES-1 and ARIES-2 trials. In another study (ARIES-3) done to evaluate the efficacy and safety of ambrisentan in patients with various PAH etiologies, a total of 224 patients with PH due to IPAH and FPAH (31%), connective tissue disease (18%), chronic hypoxemia (22%), chronic thromboembolic disease (13%), or other etiologies (16%) were enrolled, and 53% of patients received stable background PAH therapies. After 24 weeks of therapy, an increase in 6MWD (+21 m; 95% CI, 12-29) and a decrease in B-type natriuretic peptide (-26%; 95% CI, -34 to -16%) were observed in the overall population compared to baseline; however, increases in 6MWD were not observed in several non-Group 1 PH subpopulations (**Figure 7.6**).[26] Peripheral edema, headache, and dyspnea were the most common adverse events.

FIGURE 7.6 — Mean Change From Baseline in 6MWD Through Week 24 in ARIES-E

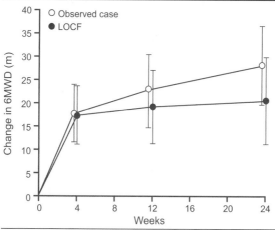

Badesch DB, et al. *Cardiovasc Ther.* 2012;30(2):93-99.

Ambrisentan dosing and monitoring information is shown in **Table 7.3**.

Macitentan

Macitentan is a tissue-targeting ET receptor blocker that inhibits binding of ET-1 to receptors ET-A and ET-B that has been FDA approved for NYHA class II-III PAH. Macitentan is a lipophilic sulfamide compound designed to decrease vascular resistance by exhibiting enhanced tissue penetration and prolonged receptor binding to ET-A/ET-B in pulmonary arterial smooth muscle cells.[27]

A long-term randomized, controlled study (Study with an Endothelin Receptor Antagonist in Pulmonary Arterial Hypertension to Improve Clinical Outcome

TABLE 7.3 — Ambrisentan Dosing and Monitoring Information

Dosing interval	Once daily
Starting dose	5 mg
Usual dose	10 mg if starting dose is tolerated
Renal impairment adjustment	Mild to moderate: none
	Severe: studies not done
Hepatic impairment dose adjustment	Mild: none
	Moderate to severe: not recommended
LFT monitoring schedule	Liver aminotransferase levels at baseline then follow clinically
When to discontinue	Discontinue ambrisentan if aminotransferase elevations are $>5 \times$ ULN or if elevations are accompanied by bilirubin $>2 \times$ ULN or by signs or symptoms of liver dysfunction, and other causes are excluded
Adverse reactions	Fluid retention
	Pulmonary edema with PVOD
	Decreased sperm count
	Hematologic changes

Letairis [package insert]. Foster City, CA: Gilead Sciences, Inc; October 2015.

[SERAPHIN]) was conducted. The study was intended to determine safety and efficacy as assessed by the time to the first occurrence of a composite endpoint of clinical worsening defined as death, atrial septostomy, lung transplantation, initiation of treatment with parenteral prostanoids, or clinical worsening. There were 250 patients assigned to placebo, 250 patients to macitentan 3 mg once daily, and 242 to macitentan 10 mg daily. Patients were treated for up to 42 months, and the median treatment period was 115 weeks. Macitentan, at both the 3-mg and 10-mg doses, decreased the risk of clinical worsening vs placebo (**Figure 7.7**).[28]

This risk was found to be reduced by 45% in the 10-mg group ($P<0.0001$), and the 3-mg group showed a risk reduction of 30% ($P=0.01$). Secondary endpoints included 6MWD change in the first 6 months of therapy as well as NYHA functional class and time to either death or hospitalization due to PAH. These endpoints also showed a dose-dependent effect ($P<0.05$ for either dose).[28]

Adverse events and discontinuation of treatment due to adverse events was similar across all groups. Adverse events associated with macitentan were headache, nasopharyngitis, and anemia. Elevations of liver aminotransferases greater than 3 times the upper limit of normal were observed in 4.5% of patients receiving

FIGURE 7.7 — Effect of Macitentan on the Composite Primary Endpoint of a First Event Related to PAH or Death From Any Cause

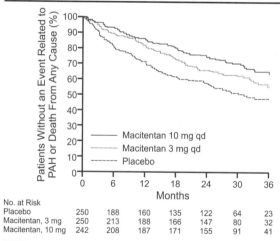

No. at Risk						
	0	6	12	18	24	30	36
Placebo	250	188	160	135	122	64	23
Macitentan, 3 mg	250	213	188	166	147	80	32
Macitentan, 10 mg	242	208	187	171	155	91	41

Worsening of PAH, initiation of treatment with IV or SC prostanoids, lung transplantation, or atrial septostomy.

Pulido T, et al. *N Engl J Med.* 2013;369:809-818.

placebo, in 3.6% of patients on 3 mg of macitentan, and in 3.4% of patients on 10 mg of macitentan.[28]

The dosing and monitoring information for macitentan are shown in **Table 7.4**.

Adverse Effects

The most frequently occurring serious adverse events with the use of ET receptor antagonists are peripheral edema, due to their vasodilatory effects, and

TABLE 7.4 — Macitentan Dosing and Monitoring Information

Dosing interval	Once daily
Starting dose	10 mg
Usual dose	10 mg
Renal impairment adjustment	None
Hepatic impairment dose adjustment	None
LFT monitoring schedule	Liver aminotransferase levels at baseline then follow clinically
When to discontinue	If clinically relevant aminotransferase elevations occur or if elevations are accompanied by an increase in bilirubin $>2 \times$ ULN, or by clinical symptoms of hepatotoxicity
Adverse reactions	Anemia
	Nasopharyngitis/pharyngitis
	Bronchitis
	Headache
	Influenza
	Urinary tract infection

Opsumit [package insert]. South San Francisco, CA: Actelion Pharmaceuticals US, Inc; April 2015.

elevation of liver aminotransferases.[20,21] Peripheral edema occurs in up to 17% of patients. Some patients may be managed with diuretics; however, more serious cases may require discontinuation of medication.

The rate of liver enzyme elevation varies among drugs in this group and mild elevations in aminotransferase levels occur only in a minority of patients. Bosentan, the first available of the ERAs, has the greatest incidence of liver enzyme elevations, and patients taking this medication require monthly monitoring of liver function tests, as has been mandated by the FDA.[20] Hepatotoxicity is uncommon with ambrisentan and macitentan, and routine monitoring in these patients is not required, but patients should be assessed for their risk of liver toxicity.[28,29] Patients at increased risk of liver dysfunction may warrant monitoring of LFTs every 3 to 4 months.

The cytochrome P450 pathways are involved in the metabolism of the ERAs more so with bosentan and macitentan. In general, ambrisentan is primarily metabolized through hepatic glucuronidation, with a minor route through the cytochrome P450 system. There is less interaction with cytochrome P450, and ambrisentan has less interaction with other medications. These characteristics confer a lower risk of drug-drug interactions with ambrisentan compared with bosentan and macitentan. The drug interactions associated with ERAs are of special interest because many of these interactions are with medications that are taken for treatment of concurrent illnesses. The use of some of these drugs is associated with potential drug-drug interactions as identified in the **Table 7.5** and **Table 7.6**.

All ERAs are potential teratogens and are considered a pregnancy category X. Women of childbearing age should have pregnancy excluded before starting treatment and should be monitored monthly while on therapy. In addition, double barrier method contraception should be utilized. Due to the teratogenic effects of ERAs, they are all part of a specially designed program enacted by the FDA called the Approved Risk

7

TABLE 7.5 — Pharmacokinetic Interactions Between ERAs and Other PAH-Specific Medications

ERA	PAH-Specific Medication	Interaction
Ambrisentan	Sildenafil/tadalafil	No interaction
Bosentan	Sildenafil	Reduces sildenafil plasma concentrations 63%. Bosentan will decrease the level or effect of sildenafil by affecting hepatic/intestinal enzyme CYP3A4 metabolism. Possible serious or life-threatening interaction. Use alternatives if available. Potent CYP3A4 inducers are expected to cause substantial decreases in sildenafil plasma levels
	Tadalafil	Reduces tadalafil Cmax 27% at steady state. Bosentan will decrease the level or effect of tadalafil by affecting hepatic/intestinal CYP3A4 metabolism. Potential for interaction; monitor
Macitentan	Sildenafil	Macitentan increases levels of sildenafil by unspecified interaction mechanism. Minor or nonsignificant interaction. Systemic exposure of steady-state sildenafil (20 mg TID) increased by 15% during coadministration of macitentan (10 mg/day); this change is not considered clinically relevant
	Tadalafil	No interaction

Letairis [package insert]. Foster City, CA: Gilead Sciences, Inc; October 2015; Tracleer [package insert]. South San Francisco, CA: Actelion Pharmaceuticals US, Inc; October 2015; Opsumit [package insert]. South San Francisco, CA: Actelion Pharmaceuticals US, Inc; April 2015; Center for Drug Evaluation and Research. Clinical Pharmacology and Biopharmaceutic Review(s). Application number 22-332. Adcirca Tablets. July 23, 2008.

TABLE 7.6 — Potential Interactions Between PAH-Specific Medications for Concurrent Illnesses

Drug	Anticoagulants	Statins	Digoxin	NSAIDs	RTIs	Protease Inhibitors	Antifungals
Bosentan	X	X	—	—	X	X	X
Ambrisentan	—	—	—	—	—	—	—
Macitentan	—	—	—	—	—	X	X

Key: X = known interaction; — = no known interaction or not clinically significant interaction.

Letairis [package insert]. Foster City, CA: Gilead Sciences, Inc; October 2015; Tracleer [package insert]. South San Francisco, CA: Actelion Pharmaceuticals US, Inc; October 2015; Opsumit [package insert]. South San Francisco, CA: Actelion Pharmaceuticals US, Inc; April 2015; Ghofrany HA, et al. *Eur Cardiol Rev.* 2009;5(1):46-51.

7

Evaluation and Mitigation Strategies (REMS). This allows the FDA to ensure from manufacturers that the benefits of a drug or biological product outweigh its risks.

Ambrisentan, bosentan, and macitentan have all been approved for the treatment of WHO Group 1 PAH patients in NYHA functional class II to IV. These medications have been shown to be effective when taken orally and have shown improvement in exercise tolerance, as well as measures of dyspnea and health-related quality of life. They are generally well tolerated and require only once or twice a day dosing. Careful consideration should be given to interactions with concomitant medications as well as liver toxicity.

Key Points

- Endothelin-1 (ET-1) is a 21-amino acid peptide produced in the endothelium that has potent vasoconstrictor properties and plays a major role in pulmonary vascular hemodynamics. It is also a culprit in vascular diseases of several organ systems, including the heart, general circulation, and the pulmonary vascular system.
- Endothelin receptor antagonists (ERAs) are indicated for treatment of WHO Group 1 PAH.
- All three ERAs that are currently available have been shown to increase exercise tolerance and delay time to clinical worsening in patients with PAH.
- Monthly monitoring of LFTs is mandatory for patients being treated with bosentan, and less frequent LFT monitoring may be indicated in patients at increased risk of liver disease in patients taking ambrisentan or macitentan.
- ERAs are potential teratogens and women of childbearing age need to use effective birth control and be monitored monthly for pregnancy.

REFERENCES

1. Agapitov AV, Haynes WG. Role of endothelin in cardiovascular disease. *J Renin Angiotensin Aldosterone Syst*. 2002;3(1):1-15.

2. Yoshimoto S, Ishizaki Y, Sasaki T, Murota S. Effect of carbon dioxide and oxygen on endothelin production by cultured porcine cerebral endothelial cells. *Stroke*. 1991;22(3):378-383.

3. Takuwa Y, Kasuya Y, Takuwa N, et al. Endothelin receptor is coupled to phospholipase C via a pertussis toxin-insensitive guanine nucleotide-binding regulatory protein in vascular smooth muscle cells. *J Clin Invest*. 1990;85(3):653-658.

4. Giaid A, Yanagisawa M, Langleben D, et al. Expression of endothelin-1 in the lungs of patients with pulmonary hypertension. *N Engl J Med*. 1993;328(24):1732-1739.

5. Dupuis J, Hoeper MM. Endothelin receptor antagonists in pulmonary arterial hypertension. *Eur Respir J*. 2008;31(2):407-415.

6. Chua BH, Krebs CJ, Chua CC, Diglio CA. Endothelin stimulates protein synthesis in smooth muscle cells. *Am J Physiol*. 1992;262(4 Pt 1):E412-E416.

7. Masaki T. Possible role of endothelin in endothelial regulation of vascular tone. *Annu Rev Pharmacol Toxicol*. 1995;35:235-255.

8. Macarthur H, Warner TD, Wood EG, Corder R, Vane JR. Endothelin-1 release from endothelial cells in culture is elevated both acutely and chronically by short periods of mechanical stretch. *Biochem Biophys Res Commun*. 1994;200(1):395-400.

9. Wesson DE, Simoni J, Green DF. Reduced extracellular pH increases endothelin-1 secretion by human renal microvascular endothelial cells. *J Clin Invest*. 1998;101(3):578-583.

10. Rakugi H, Tabuchi Y, Nakamaru M, et al. Evidence for endothelin-1 release from resistance vessels of rats in response to hypoxia. *Biochem Biophys Res Commun*. 1990;169(3):973-977.

11. Imai T, Hirata Y, Emori T, Yanagisawa M, Masaki T, Marumo F. Induction of endothelin-1 gene by angiotensin and vasopressin in endothelial cells. *Hypertension*. 1992;19(6 Pt 2):753-757.

12. Matsuura A, Yamochi W, Hirata K, Kawashima S, Yokoyama M. Stimulatory interaction between vascular endothelial growth factor and endothelin-1 on each gene expression. *Hypertension*. 1998;32(1):89-95.

13. Schwarting A, Schlaak J, Lotz J, Pfers I, Meyer zum Büschenfelde KH, Mayet WJ. Endothelin-1 modulates the expression

of adhesion molecules on fibroblast-like synovial cells (FLS). *Scand J Rheumatol.* 1996;25(4):246-256.

14. Boulanger C, Lüscher TF. Release of endothelin from the porcine aorta. Inhibition by endothelium-derived nitric oxide. *J Clin Invest.* 1990;85(2):587-590.

15. Stewart DJ, Cernacek P, Mohamed F, Blais D, Cianflone K, Monge JC. Role of cyclic nucleotides in the regulation of endothelin-1 production by human endothelial cells. *Am J Physiol.* 1994;266(3 Pt 2):H944-H951.

16. Morey AK, Razandi M, Pedram A, Hu RM, Prins BA, Levin ER. Oestrogen and progesterone inhibit the stimulated production of endothelin-1. *Biochem J.* 1998;330 (Pt 3):1097-1105.

17. Chen SJ, Chen YF, Meng QC, Durand J, Dicarlo VS, Oparil S. Endothelin-receptor antagonist bosentan prevents and reverses hypoxic pulmonary hypertension in rats. *J Appl Physiol (1985).* 1995;79(6):2122-2131.

18. Williamson DJ, Wallman LL, Jones R, et al. Hemodynamic effects of Bosentan, an endothelin receptor antagonist, in patients with pulmonary hypertension. *Circulation.* 2000;102(4):411-418.

19. Channick RN, Simonneau G, Sitbon O, et al. Effects of the dual endothelin-receptor antagonist bosentan in patients with pulmonary hypertension: a randomised placebo-controlled study. *Lancet.* 2001;358(9288):1119-1123.

20. Rubin LJ, Badesch DB, Barst RJ, et al. Bosentan therapy for pulmonary arterial hypertension. *N Engl J Med.* 2002;346(12):896-903.

21. Galiè N, Rubin Lj, Hoeper M, et al. Treatment of patients with mildly symptomatic pulmonary arterial hypertension with bosentan (EARLY study): a double-blind, randomised controlled trial. *Lancet.* 2008;371(9630):2093-2100.

22. Galiè N, Beghetti M, Gatzoulis MA et al; Bosentan Randomized Trial of Endothelin Antagonist Therapy-5 (BREATHE-5) Investigators. Bosentan therapy in patients with Eisenmenger syndrome: a multicenter, double-blind, randomized, placebo-controlled study. *Circulation.* 2006;114(1):48-54.

23. Opitz CF, Ewert R, Kirch W, Pittrow D. Inhibition of endothelin receptors in the treatment of pulmonary arterial hypertension: does selectivity matter? *Eur Heart J.* 2008;29(16):1936-1948.

24. Galié N, Badesch D, Oudiz R, et al. Ambrisentan therapy for pulmonary arterial hypertension. *J Am Coll Cardiol.* 2005;46(3):529-535.

25. Galiè N, Olschewski H, Oudiz RJ, et al; Ambrisentan in Pulmonary Arterial Hypertension, Randomized, Double-Blind, Placebo-Controlled, Multicenter, Efficacy Studies (ARIES) Group. Ambrisentan for the treatment of pulmonary arterial hypertension: results of the ambrisentan in pulmonary arterial hypertension, randomized, double-blind, placebo-controlled, multicenter, efficacy (ARIES) study 1 and 2. *Circulation*. 2008;117(23):3010-3019.

26. Badesch DB, Feldman J, Keogh A, et al; ARIES-3 Study Group. ARIES-3: ambrisentan therapy in a diverse population of patients with pulmonary hypertension. *Cardiovasc Ther*. 2012;30(2):93-99.

27. Iglarz M, Binkert C, Morrison K, et al. Pharmacology of macitentan, an orally active tissue-targeting dual endothelin receptor antagonist. *J Pharmacol Exp Ther*. 2008;327(3):736-745.

28. Pulido T, Adzerikho I, Channick RN, et al; SERAPHIN Investigators. Macitentan and morbidity and mortality in pulmonary arterial hypertension. *N Engl J Med*. 2013;369(9):809-818.

29. Oudiz RJ, Galiè N, Olschewski H, et al; ARIES Study Group. Long-term ambrisentan therapy for the treatment of pulmonary arterial hypertension. *J Am Coll Cardiol*. 2009;54(21):1971-1981.

7

8

Phosphodiesterase-5 Inhibitors

by James R. Klinger, MD

Mechanism of Action

The cyclic nucleotides cAMP and cGMP play important roles in modulating vascular smooth muscle tone. Most of the vasodilating properties of NO and the natriuretic peptides are mediated via activation of guanylate cyclases that convert 5′ mono GTP to cGMP and thereby increase intracellular cGMP levels (**Figure 8.1**). In turn, cGMP is capable of activating cGMP-dependent protein kinase (PKG) that acts at multiple downstream targets to decrease intracellular calcium $[Ca^{2+}]_i$.[1] PKG can also relax vascular smooth muscle by inhibiting myosin light chain phosphatase and by phosphorylating myosin-binding proteins.[2] cGMP is also capable of directly activating cGMP-gated cation channels to block Ca^{++} entry into cells. In addition to its effect on decreasing $[Ca^{2+}]_i$, cGMP has antiproliferative effects that help mitigate pulmonary vascular remodeling.

Intracellular cGMP levels are determined by the rates of cGMP synthesis and degradation. Pulmonary vascular cGMP is synthesized via activation of soluble guanylate cyclase (sGC) by NO and particulate guanylate cyclases (pGC) by natriuretic peptides (**Figure 8.1**). NO is synthesized in vascular endothelial cells from L-arginine and oxygen by endothelial nitric oxide synthase (eNOS) and diffuses into adjacent smooth muscle cells and binds to sGC. Atrial and brain natriuretic peptide (ANP, BNP) are synthesized in the cardiac atria and ventricles and are released in response to increases in intrachamber pressure or volume loading.

FIGURE 8.1 — Role of Intracellular cGMP in the Modulation of Pulmonary Vascular Smooth Muscle Relaxation

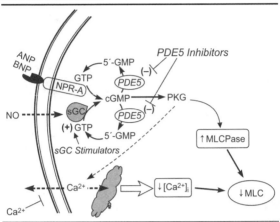

Intracellular cGMP is synthesized from GTP via activation of soluble guanylate cyclase (sGC) by nitric oxide (NO) or via activation of the particulate guanylate cyclase-linked cell surface receptor, natriuretic peptide receptor-A (NPR-A), by ANP or BNP. cGMP activates protein kinase G (PKG) which acts through a variety of mechanisms to decrease intracellular calcium $[Ca^{2+}]_i$ and increase myosin light chain phosphotase (MLCPase) leading to decreased phosphorylation of myosin light chain (MLC) and smooth muscle relaxation.

C-type natriuretic peptide (CNP) is synthesized by vascular endothelial cells. Natriuretic peptides released by the right heart or by pulmonary vascular endothelial cells activate pGCs on the cell surface of pulmonary vascular smooth muscle. Two types of pGCs with high affinity for the natriuretic peptides have been described. Natriuretic peptide receptor-A (NPR-A) has high binding affinity for ANP and BNP. Natriuretic peptide receptor-B (NPR-B) has high binding affinity for C-type natriuretic peptide (CNP). Increasing pulmonary vascular cGMP levels via administration of NO, natriuretic peptides, or sGCs stimulators have been shown to mitigate PH and right ventricular hypertrophic changes in animal models of PH.[3-6] Furthermore, mice with targeted deletion of the genes for endothelial nitric oxide synthase (eNOS), ANP, or NPR-A develop more severe PH when exposed to chronic hypoxia.[7-9]

Phosphodiesterase Inhibitors

Newly synthesized cGMP is metabolized primarily by degradation via phosphodiesterases (PDEs). Over a dozen PDEs have been identified with various degrees of activity for cGMP and cAMP. The PDEs that are most responsible for cGMP in the pulmonary circulation is the type-2 and type-5 isoform (PDE2, PDE5).[10,11] Several lines of evidence suggest that pulmonary vascular endothelial NO and natriuretic peptide signaling are impaired in PAH.[10,11] At the same time, increased activity of PDE5 has been demonstrated in some animal models of PH.[12,13] Together, these findings are likely to result in decreased intracellular cGMP levels in patients with PAH.

The acute pulmonary vasodilator effects of NO and the natriuretic peptides are potentiated by inhibition of PDE. This is particularly true for inhibitors of PDE5 and PDE2. Degradation by PDE5 is also the primary metabolic route of cGMP in the corpus cavernosum. Three PDE5 inhibitors have been developed and approved for the treatment of male erectile dysfunction based on their ability to delay cGMP metabolism and enhance vasodilation during penile erection. All three drugs have subsequently been studied for the treatment of PAH based on the high concentration of PDE5 in lung (**Figure 8**.2). Two of these, sildenafil and tadalafil, are presently approved for PAH treatment in the United States.

FIGURE 8.2 — Change in Pulmonary Vascular Resistance in Response to Phosphodiesterase Inhibitors

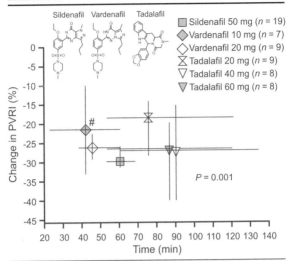

Point estimates of median differences in percentage of baseline pulmonary vascular resistance index with 95% CIs represented by vertical bars following a single dose of the three currently available phosphodiesterase inhibitors in the United States. Although peak vasodilator response occurred later with tadalafil than with vardenafil ($P<0.001$), there was no difference in the magnitude of response among the treatment groups ($P=0.185$ for vardenafil 20 mg vs sildenafil 50 mg, vs tadalafil 40 mg).

Adapted from Ghofrani HA, et al. *J Am Coll Cardiol.* 2004;44(7): 1488-1496.

Sildenafil and Tadalafil for Treatment of PAH

Case reports and small case series of PAH patients responding favorably to sildenafil began to appear in the literature around 2000. Several animal studies showing attenuation of monocrotaline and hypoxia-induced PH in animals contributed to the hypothesis that pulmonary hypertension could be mitigated by inhibiting cGMP metabolism. Shortly thereafter, sildenafil was approved by the FDA for the treatment of PAH based primarily on the results of the SUPER trial,[14] a large placebo-controlled study that randomized 278 treatment-naïve patients to placebo or 20, 40, or 80 mg of sildenafil 3 times daily for 12 weeks. The primary outcome measure of placebo-adjusted increased in 6MWD was reached for all three treatment groups, but there was no significant difference in treatment effect between the three sildenafil doses studied (**Figure 8.3**) and the drug was approved at the 20-mg dose.

At about the same time that sildenafil was approved, several investigators reported favorable effects of tadalafil for the treatment of PAH. Its longer half-life and once-daily dosing generated interest in its use as a long-term therapy for PAH and a phase 3 clinical trial was organized. Tadalafil was approved for treatment of PAH in the United States in 2009 based on data from the PHIRST-1 study that randomized 405 PAH patients to placebo or tadalafil at 2.5, 10, 20, or 40 mg once daily for 16 weeks.[15] Approximately half of the patients in the study were treatment-naïve and the other half had background therapy with an endothelin receptor antagonist that was continued during the study. The primary outcome measure was placebo-adjusted increase in 6MWD after 16 weeks of treatment and was met only in patients in the highest treatment dose group (**Figure 8.3**). Tadalafil was subsequently approved for treatment of PAH at the dose of 40 mg per day.

Effect of Sildenafil and Tadalafil on Exercise Capacity

The mean increase in 6MWD achieved with sildenafil and tadalafil is likely to be clinically significant. Recent studies suggest that 38.6 meters is the minimal important difference (MID) in 6MWD for patients with PAH.[16] The mean increase in 6MWD was 45 meters

FIGURE 8.3 — Change in 6MWD in Pivotal Clinical Trials of Sildenafil and Tadalafil

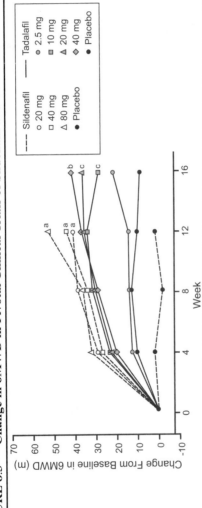

Change in 6MWD from baseline for each placebo and treatment group in the pivotal clinical trials of sildenafil (SUPER study) and tadalafil (PHIRST study) for PAH. Values shown are mean. $N = 67$-71 for each sildenafil-treatment group and 78-82 for each tadalafil-treatment group. [a] $P < 0.001$, [b] $P < 0.01$, [c] $P < 0.05$ vs placebo. Patients in the sildenafil trial were treatment-naïve; approximately half of those enrolled in the tadalafil study were already taking bosentan at time of study entry.

Modified from Galie N, et al. *N Engl J Med.* 2005;353(20):2148-2157; Galie N, et al. *Circulation.* 2009;119(22):2894-2903.

for the 20-mg sildenafil-treatment group in the SUPER study and 33 meters for the 40-mg tadalafil-treatment group in the PHIRST-1 study (**Figure 8.3**).[14,15] Treatment-naïve patients treated with the 40-mg dose of tadalafil in PHIRST-1 had a 44 meter improvement in 6MWD.[15] Together, these studies strongly suggest that PDE5 inhibitors improve functional capacity as assessed by 6MWD in treatment-naïve patients with PAH for at least the first 3 to 4 months of therapy.

Hemodynamic Effects

Pulmonary hemodynamics were measured at baseline and after 12 weeks of treatment in all patients who participated in the SUPER trial.[14] Compared with placebo, mPAP and PVR were lower in patients who received any of the three doses of sildenafil. In patients assigned to the 20-mg treatment dose, mean PA pressure and the PVR decreased -2.1 mm Hg (95% CI, -4.3 to 0.0; $P=0.04$) and -122 dyn·sec·cm^{-5} (95% CI, -217 to -27; $P=0.01$), respectively. There was a strong trend toward an increase in cardiac index (0.21 L/min per square meter, 95% CI, 0.04 to 0.8; $P=0.06$). Greater hemodynamic improvement was seen in patients who received 80 mg tid vs 20 mg tid.

Right heart catheterization was performed at baseline and after 16 weeks of treatment in 93 patients treated with 20 or 40 mg of tadalafil in the PHIRST study.[15] The mPAP and the PVR decreased -4.3 mm Hg (95% CI, -8 to -1; $P=0.01$) and -209 dyn·sec·cm^{-5} (95% CI, -406 to -13; $P=0.039$), respectively, in patients assigned to the 40-mg dose. Cardiac index also increased 0.6 L/min per square meter (95% CI, 0.1 to 1.6; $n=18$, $P=0.028$).

The significant decrease in both mPAP and PVR for the 20-mg sildenafil treatment group and the 40-mg tadalafil treatment group strongly suggest that PDE5 inhibitors are capable of improving pulmonary hemodynamics at the currently approved treatment dose over the first few months of therapy in patients with PAH.

Effect on Functional Class and Time to Clinical Worsening

The proportion of patients who improved at least one WHO functional class in the SUPER study was significantly greater in each sildenafil-treatment group than in the placebo group.[14] Only 7% of patients treated with placebo improved their functional class compared with 28%, 36%, and 42% of patients treated with 20, 40, and 80 mg tid of sildenafil, respectively. Although the proportion of patients who increased or decreased at least one WHO functional class was not significantly different between placebo or any of the four treatment groups that received tadalafil in the PHIRST-1 study, approximately half of each cohort had been on background therapy for an average of nearly a year before study entry. A post hoc analysis of patients who were treatment-naïve found that 38% of patients in the 40-mg tadalafil group improved at least one WHO functional class during 16 weeks of therapy vs only 16% of patients in the placebo group ($P=0.03$).[15]

Patients treated with 40 mg daily of tadalafil in the PHIRST trial had a delay in time to clinical worsening and a lower incidence of clinical worsening than patients treated with placebo.[15] No difference in time to clinical worsening or the incidence of clinical worsening was seen between placebo and any dose of sildenafil in the SUPER study. However, it should be noted that the lower incidence of clinical worsening in the tadalafil study was driven almost entirely by a lower proportion of patients who declined at least one WHO functional class, and this metric was not included in the definition of clinical worsening in the sildenafil study.

Long-Term Effect of PDE5 Inhibitors

Limited data are available regarding the efficacy of long-term treatment of PAH with PDE5 inhibitors. Both the SUPER and PHIRST-1 studies had long-term follow-up arms showing that the improvement in the primary outcome measure (6MWD) observed after 12 to 16 weeks of treatment were maintained up to a year with both sildenafil and tadalafil.[14,15]

In the SUPER study, patients who elected to stay in the longer-term extension study were increased to 80 mg 3 times daily, and those who remained on monotherapy (222 of the 259 who elected to participate in the extension) maintained their increase in 6MWD for 1 year (48 meters at 12 weeks vs 51 meters at 12 months). The durability of treatment effect on 6MWD or hemodynamics for the currently approved 20-mg dose of sildenafil has not been studied.

In the PHIRST-1 study, 213 of 357 patients (60%) enrolled in the extension study had received tadalafil for at least 10 months at the time of publication. Their improvement in 6MWD was 37 meters at 16 weeks (95% CI, 30-44) and 38 meters after 44 weeks (95% CI, 29-47).

Adverse Effects of PDE5 Inhibitors

In general, PDE5 inhibitors have been well tolerated in patients with PAH. The most common adverse effects are headache, flushing, epistaxis, dyspepsia, and myalgias including back pain.[14,15] Serious adverse events were reported in 25% and 13% of patients in the SUPER and PHIRST trials (**Table 8.1**), but were judged by the investigators to be drug related in less than 3% of cases. In a post hoc analysis of the PHIRST trial, the incidence of adverse events in patients given 40-mg tadalafil was no different in patients >65 years of age compared with those who were <65 years old.[17]

Rare cases of vascular thrombosis have been reported following the use of PDE5 inhibitors including a case of acute PE associated with sildenafil in the SUPER trial and associated with tadalafil use in a patient with protein C deficiency.[18] There may also be a relationship between PDE5 inhibitors and nonarteritic ischemic optic neuropathy (NAION). Although the

TABLE 8.1 — Most Frequent Adverse Events Reported by Patients in the SUPER and PHIRST Trials[a]

	n	Headache	Diarrhea	Back Pain	Dyspepsia	Flushing	Myalgia	Limb Pain	Epistaxis	Insomnia	Visual Disturbance
Placebo	70	27	6	11	7	4	4	6	1	1	0
Sildenafil 20 mg tid	69	32	9	13	13	10	7	7	9	7	0
Sildenafil 40 mg tid	67	28	12	13	9	9	6	15	7	6	4
Sildenafil 80 mg tid	71	35	10	8	13	15	14	8	4	4	7
Placebo	82	15	10	6	2	2	4	2	4	2	1
Tadalafil 2.5 mg qd	82	18	11	6	5	4	2	4	7	2	2
Tadalafil 10 mg qd	80	38	11	6	3	6	4	5	5	1	3
Tadalafil 20 mg qd	82	32	7	12	13	6	9	5	6	5	5
Tadalafil 40 mg qd	79	42	11	10	10	13	14	11	4	4	3

[a] Adverse events listed are those reported by 3% of patients and those that were reported more frequently in the treated group than in the placebo group.

Galie N, et al. *N Engl J Med*. 2005;353:2148-2157; Galie N, et al. *Circulation*. 2009;11:2894-2903.

number of cases has been too low to directly link the use of PDE5 inhibitors with NAION, several reports have raised the possibility of this association with sildenafil and with tadalafil when taken for erectile dysfunction.[19,20] Patients who develop a change in vision while taking a PDE5 inhibitor should discontinue the drug and undergo ophthalmologic consultation.

Sildenafil and tadalafil are absorbed rapidly, reaching peak plasma concentrations approximately 1 and 2 hours after ingestion, respectively, and are metabolized primarily in the liver via cytochrome P450 (CYP). Sildenafil is metabolized primarily by CYP3A4 with minor contribution from CYP2C9 and CPY2C19. Tadalafil is metabolized primarily by CYP3A4. Plasma elimination half-life is approximately 4 hours for sildenafil and 17.5 hours for tadalafil in healthy volunteers but may be considerably longer in patients with PAH. Due to its hepatic and renal routes of elimination, it is advisable to start tadalafil at no more than 20 mg a day in patients with mild to moderate hepatic or renal disease and increase to 40 mg daily based on individual tolerability. Tadalafil should be avoided in patients with more severe liver or renal impairment.

All PDE5 inhibitors should not be used with nitrates due to the potential for hypotension and coronary ischemia. Potent inhibitors of CYP3A such as itraconazole, ketoconazole, or ritonavir should be avoided as they may prolong the metabolism of sildenafil or tadalafil. Patients with PAH associated with HIV infection who are taking ritonavir may tolerate 20 mg of tadalafil better than the approved dose of 40 mg qd.

Recommendations For Use

Sildenafil and tadalafil are approved for treatment of WHO Group 1 PAH patients in WHO functional class II or III. These agents appear to be as effective as other orally active medications at improving 6MWD and WHO functional class, decreasing PVR, and slowing time to clinical worsening. In addition, they are generally well tolerated, require no regular laboratory monitoring, and are considerably less expensive than other currently approved treatments for PAH. Sildenafil is also available in generic form. These characteristics make PDE5 inhibitors attractive agents for the initial treatment of PAH and are responsible for their rapid growth in the management of this disease.

Key Points

- cGMP mediates the pulmonary vasodilator and antimitogenic effects of NO and the natriuretic peptides.
- In the lung, cGMP is synthesized by activation of soluble and particulate guanylate cyclases via nitric oxide and the natriuretic peptides, respectively.
- cGMP is metabolized primarily by phosphodiesterase type-5 and inhibition of this enzyme increases intracellular cGMP levels.
- Phosphodiesterase type-5 inhibitors have been shown to improve functional capacity and pulmonary hemodynamics and delay time to clinical worsening in patients with PAH.

1. Lincoln TM, Dey N, Sellak H. Invited review: cGMP-dependent protein kinase signaling mechanisms in smooth muscle: from the regulation of tone to gene expression. *J Appl Physiol*. 2001;91:1421-1430.

2. Surks HK, Mochizuki N, Kasai Y, et al: Regulation of myosin phosphatase by a specific interaction with cGMP-dependent protein kinase I alpha. *Science*. 1999;286(5444):1583-1587.

3. Frostell CG, Blomqvist H, Hedenstierna G, Lundberg J, Zapol WM. Inhaled nitric oxide selectively reverses human hypoxic pulmonary vasoconstriction without causing systemic vasodilation. *Anesthesiology*. 1993;78(3):427-435.

4. Wanstall JC, Hughes IE, O'Donnell SR. Evidence that nitric oxide from the endothelium attenuates inherent tone in isolated pulmonary arteries from rats with hypoxic pulmonary hypertension. *Br J Pharmacol*. 1995;114(1):109-114.

5. Hill NS, Klinger JR, Warburton RR, Pietras L, Wrenn DS. Brain natriuretic peptide: possible role in the modulation of hypoxic pulmonary hypertension. *Am J Physiol*. 1994;266(3 Pt 1):L308-L315.

6. Jin H, Yang RH, Chen YF, Jackson RM, Oparil S. Atrial natriuretic peptide attenuates the development of pulmonary hypertension in rats adapted to chronic hypoxia. *J Clin Invest*. 1990;85(1):115-120.

7. Klinger JR, Warburton RR, Pietras L, et al. Targeted disruption of the gene for natriuretic peptide receptor-A worsens hypoxia-induced cardiac hypertrophy. *Am J Physiol Heart Circ Physiol*. 2002;282(1):H58-H65.

8. Zhao L, Long L, Morrell NW, Wilkins MR. NPR-A-Deficient mice show increased susceptibility to hypoxia-induced pulmonary hypertension. *Circulation*. 1999;99(5):605-607.

9. Fagan KA, Fouty BW, Tyler RC, et al. The pulmonary circulation of homozygous or heterozygous eNOS-null mice is hyperresponsive to mild hypoxia. *J Clin Invest*. 1999;103(2):291-299.

10. Lugnier C. Cyclic nucleotide phosphodiesterase (PDE) superfamily: a new target for the development of specific therapeutic agents. *Pharmacol Ther*. 2006;109(3):366-398.

11. Keravis T, Lugnier C. Cyclic nucleotide phosphodiesterases (PDE) and peptide motifs. *Curr Pharm Des*. 2010;16(9):1114-1125.

8

12. Maclean MR, Johnston ED, Mcculloch KM, Pooley L, Houslay MD, Sweeney G. Phosphodiesterase isoforms in the pulmonary arterial circulation of the rat: changes in pulmonary hypertension. *J Pharmacol Exp Ther*. 1997;283(2):619-624.

13. Hanson KA, Ziegler JW, Rybalkin SD, Miller JW, Abman SH, Clarke WR. Chronic pulmonary hypertension increases fetal lung cGMP phosphodiesterase activity. *Am J Physiol*. 1998;275:L931-L941.

14. Galie N, Ghofrani HA, Torbicki A, et al. Sildenafil citrate therapy for pulmonary arterial hypertension. *N Engl J Med*. 2005;353(20):2148-2157.

15. Galie N, Brundage BH, Ghofrani HA, et al. Tadalafil therapy for pulmonary arterial hypertension. *Circulation*. 2009;119(22):2894-2903.

16. Mathai SC, Puhan MA, Lam D, Wise RA. The minimal important difference in the 6-minute walk test for patients with pulmonary arterial hypertension. *Am J Respir Crit Care Med*. 2012;186(5):428-433.

17. Berman-Rosenzweig E, Arneson C, Klinger JR. Effects of dose and age on adverse events associated with tadalafil in the treatment of pulmonary arterial hypertension. *Pulm Circ*. 2014;4(1):45-52.

18. Chen HC, Wang CS, Chuang SH, Wang CY. Pulmonary embolism after tadalafil ingestion. *Pharm World Sci*. 2008;30(5):610-612.

19. Tripathi A, O'Donnell NP. Branch retinal artery occlusion; another complication of sildenafil. *Br J Ophthalmol*. 2000;84(8):934-935.

20. Bollinger K, Lee MS. Recurrent visual field defect and ischemic optic neuropathy associated with tadalafil rechallenge. *Arch Ophthalmol*. 2005;123(3):400-401.

9

Soluble Guanylate Cyclase Stimulators

*by Arunabh Talwar, MD and
Sonu Sahni, MD*

Nitric oxide (NO) in healthy individuals acts as a signaling molecule that induces vasodilation by relaxing vascular smooth muscle. NO works by binding soluble guanylate cyclase (sGC), which in turn induces the production of cGMP, a secondary messenger. Cyclic GMP then activates cGMP-dependent protein kinase (protein kinase G) to regulate cytosolic calcium ion concentration that leads to vasodilation (**Figure 9.1**).[1] In patients with PAH, NO synthesis is decreased and/or dysregulated leading to decreased availability of NO that contributes to reduced pulmonary vasodilation.

Riociguat

Riociguat (Adempas) is a direct sGC stimulator that has recently been approved by the FDA for the treatment of PAH and CTEPH (see *Chapter 11*). Riociguat has a dual mode of action, directly stimulating sGC activity independent of NO[2] and increasing the sensitivity of sGC to NO. It acts in synergy with NO to produce anti-aggregatory, antiproliferative, and vasodilatory effects[3,4] by increasing the synthesis of cGMP.

■ History

Riociguat was originally identified by Bayer Pharmaceuticals as BAY 63-2521 after numerous trials of similar compounds.[5] In preclinical trials, chronic treatment with BAY 63-2521 partially reversed PH, right heart hypertrophy, and pulmonary vascular remodeling in hypoxic mice, and in rats with MCT-

FIGURE 9.1 — The NO/cGMP Signaling Pathway

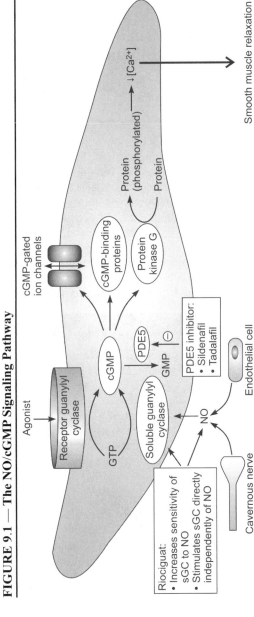

Modified from Ghofrani HA, et al. *Nat Rev Drug Discov.* 2006;5(8):689-702.

induced PH[6] phase 1 clinical trials, found that the optimal tolerated dose was 1.0 mg to 2.5 mg. At this dose, riociguat had a favorable safety profile and improved cardiac index to a greater extent than inhaled NO. However, it also had significant systemic effects and showed no pulmonary selectivity, although mean SBP remained >110 mm Hg in subjects who received it.[3]

■ Phase 2 Trials

A phase 2 trial was designed to evaluate the safety, tolerability, and efficacy of riociguat in patients with moderate-to-severe PAH and CTEPH. A total of 75 patients received at least one dose of riociguat in this 12-week, multicenter, open-label, uncontrolled study. Patients were given riociguat at a dose of 1.0 mg to 2.5 mg according to systemic SBP. Asymptomatic hypotension (SBP<90 mm Hg) occurred in 11 patients, requiring dose reduction in two patients. The median increase from baseline in 6MWD was 57 and 55 m for patients with PAH and CTEPH, respectively ($P<0.0001$).[7] PAP decreased 4.0 and 4.5 mm Hg in patients with PAH and CTEPH, respectively, and PVR decreased by 215 dyn·sec·cm^{-5} ($P<0.0001$). Dyspepsia, headache, and hypotension were the most frequent adverse events and resulted in discontinuation of drug in 4%.

■ Phase 3 Trials

Two phase 3 multicenter clinical studies were performed. One examined the efficacy of riociguat in the treatment of CTEPH and the other examined the effect of riociguat in a population of patients with PAH.

The Chronic Thromboembolic Pulmonary Hypertension sGC-Stimulator Trial (CHEST-1) was a randomized, placebo-controlled trial that enrolled 261 patients with inoperable CTEPH or persistent or recurrent PH after pulmonary endarterectomy.[8] Patients were given placebo or riociguat in individually adjusted doses of up to 2.5 mg 3 times daily. By week 16, the primary endpoint, defined as the change from baseline in the 6MWD, had increased by a mean of 39 m in the riociguat group compared with a mean decrease of 6 m in the placebo group (least-squares mean difference, 46 m; 95% CI, 25 to 67; $P<0.001$) (**Figure 9.2**). In addition, PVR decreased by 226 dyn·sec·cm^{-5} compared with an increase of 23 dyn·sec·cm^{-5} in the placebo group (least-squares mean difference, -246 dyn·sec·cm^{-5}; 95% CI, -303 to -190; $P<0.001$).[3] Riociguat was also associated with significant improvements in the NT-proBNP level ($P<0.001$), WHO functional class ($P=0.003$) (**Table 9.1**), and Borg Dyspnea Scale (**Table 9.1**). The most common serious adverse events were right ventricular failure and syncope, which were found to be comparable in both placebo and riociguat groups.

FIGURE 9.2 — CHEST-1 Study: Mean Change From Baseline in the 6MWD

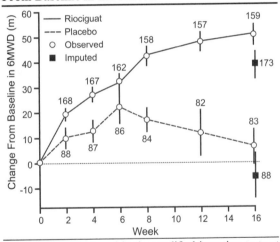

The data were analyzed in the modified intention-to-treat population without imputation of missing values; imputed values are provided at week 16. The number at each data point indicates the number of patients included in the assessment at that time point.

The least-squares mean difference in the 6MWD at week 16 was 46 m (95% CI, 25 to 67; $P<0.001$).

Ghofrani HA, et al. *N Engl J Med.* 2013;369(4):319-329.

TABLE 9.1 — CHEST-1 Study: Change From Baseline to End of Week 13 in Primary and Secondary Endpoints

Endpoint	Placebo			Riociguat		
	N	Baseline	Change	N	Baseline	Change
Primary Endpoint						
6MWD (m)	88	356±75	-6±84	173	342±82	39±79
Secondary Endpoints						
PVR (dyn·sec·cm⁻⁵)	82	779±401	23±274	151	791±432	-226±248
NT-proBNP (pg/mL)	73	1706±2567	76±1447	150	1508±2338	-291±1717
WHO functional class	87	0 patients in class I; 25 (29%) in class II, 60 (69%) in class III, 2 (2%) in class IV	13 patients (15%) moved to lower class (indicating improvement), 68 (78%) stayed in same class, 6 (7%) moved to higher class	173	3 patients (2%) in class I, 55 (32%) in class II, 107 (62%) in class III, 8 (5%) in class IV	57 patients (33%) moved to lower class (indicating improvement), 107 (62%) stayed in same class, 9 (5%) moved to higher class

Ghofrani HA, et al. *N Engl J Med*. 2013;369(4):319-329.

9

Patients who completed the initial trial were enrolled in an extension study, CHEST-2, to further determine long-term safety and efficacy.[9] In the observed population at 1 year ($n=172$), improvements in 6MWD and WHO FC were similar to those observed in CHEST-1. The mean ± SD improvement in 6MWD from baseline was +51±62 m and WHO FC had improved/stabilized/worsened in 47%/50%/3% of patients.

Another trial, the Pulmonary Arterial Hypertension sGC-Stimulator Trial (PATENT-1), was a randomized, placebo-controlled trial that investigated the efficacy and safety of riociguat in PAH patients.[10] Study eligibility included patients who were receiving no other treatment for PAH and patients who were receiving ERAs or (non-intravenous) prostanoids. Four hundred forty-three patients with symptomatic PAH were randomized to receive placebo, riociguat in individually adjusted doses of up to 2.5 mg 3 times daily (2.5 mg–maximum group), or riociguat in individually adjusted doses that were capped at 1.5 mg 3 times daily (1.5 mg–maximum group). After a 12-week treatment, the change from baseline in 6MWD had increased by a mean of 30 m in the 2.5 mg–maximum group and had decreased by a mean of 6 m in the placebo group (least-squares mean difference, 36 m; 95% CI, 20-52; $P<0.001$) (Figure 9.3).

In addition, subgroup analyses showed that riociguat improved the 6MWD both in patients who were treatment-naïve, as well as in those who were receiving ERAs or prostanoids.[10] Secondary endpoints were also evaluated and showed decreases in PVRs ($P<0.001$), NT-proBNP levels ($P<0.001$), and time to clinical worsening ($P=0.005$), and improvements in WHO functional class ($P=0.003$) and Borg dyspnea score ($P=0.002$) (Table 9.2). There was also significant improvements in mean PAP and cardiac output ($P<0.001$). The placebo group showed increased events of clinical worsening compared with the titrated group.[10] The most common serious adverse event in the placebo group and the 2.5 mg–maximum group

FIGURE 9.3 — PATENT-1 Study: Mean Change From Baseline in the 6MWD

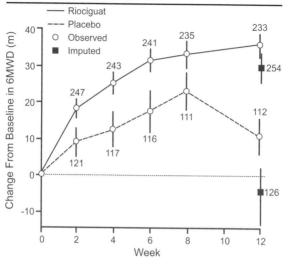

The data were analyzed in the modified intention-to-treat population without imputation of missing values; imputed values are provided at week 12. The number at each data point indicates the number of patients included in the assessment at that time point.

The least-squares mean difference in the 6MWD at week 12 was 36 m (95% CI, 20 to 52; $P<0.001$).

Ghofrani HA, et al. *N Engl J Med*. 2013;369(4):330-340.

was syncope (4% and 1%, respectively). Patients who completed the initial trial were enrolled in an extension study, PATENT-2, to evaluate longer term safety and efficacy.[11] A total of 396 of the 443 patients enrolled in PATENT entered the extension study, and 324 patients were in the study at the time of analysis. In the observed population at the 1-year time point, riociguat was well tolerated, mean±sd 6MWD had changed by 51 ± 74 m, and WHO functional class had improved/stabilized/worsened in 33%/61%/6% of patients.[11]

The dosing and monitoring information for riociguat is shown in **Table 9.3**.

TABLE 9.2 — PATENT-1 Study: Change From Baseline to End of Week 13 in Primary and Secondary Endpoints

Endpoint	Placebo			Riociguat, Maximum 2.5 mg TID		
	N	Baseline	Change	N	Baseline	Change
Primary Endpoint						
6-min walk distance	126	368±75	-6±86	254	361±68	30±66
Secondary Endpoints						
PVR (dyn·sec·cm⁻⁵)	107	834±477	-9±317	232	791±453	-223±260
NT-prBNP (pg/mL)	106	1228±1775	232±1011	228	1027±1799	-198±1721
WHO functional class	125	4 patients (3%) in class I, 60 (48%) in class II, 58 (46%) in class III, 3 (2%) in class IV	18 patients (14%) moved to lower class (indicating improvement), 89 (71%) stayed in same class, 18 (14%) moved to higher class	254	5 patients (2%) in class I, 108 (43%) in class II, 140 (55%) in class III, 1 (0.4%) in class IV	53 patients (21%) moved to lower class (indicating improvement), 192 (76%) stayed in same class, 9 (4%) moved to higher class

Ghofrani HA, et al. *N Engl J Med.* 2013;369(4):330-340.

TABLE 9.3 — Riociguat Dosing and Monitoring Information

Dosing interval	3 times daily
Starting dose	1 mg for 4 weeks (0.5 mg if patient does not tolerate hypotensive effects)
Usual dose	1 mg 3 times daily
Renal impairment adjustment	Not recommended in patients with CrCl <15 mL/min or on dialysis
Hepatic impairment dose adjustment	Mild or moderate: administer with caution
	Severe: avoid
LFT monitoring schedule	N/A
When to discontinue	No clinical experience with riociguat in patients with elevated liver aminotransferases ($>3 \times$ ULN) or with elevated direct bilirubin ($>2 \times$ ULN) prior to initiation of treatment; riociguat is not recommended in these patients
Adverse reactions	Headache
	Dyspepsia and gastritis
	Dizziness
	Nausea
	Hypotension
	Vomiting
	Anemia
	GERD
	Constipation

Adempas [package insert]. Whippany, NJ: Bayer HealthCare Pharmaceuticals Inc; September 2014.

9

■ Adverse Events/Side Effects

Generally, riociguat is well tolerated. The most common side effects are headache and dizziness, which have been seen in up to one quarter of patients. Other common side effects include upset stomach, leg swelling, runny nose, and nausea. The most frequently occurring serious adverse events in clinical trials were right ventricular failure and syncope, which were comparable to the placebo group (2% of the riociguat group). In pooled analysis of the PATENT and CHEST studies, serious hemoptysis occurred in 1% of patients taking riociguat and 0% of patients taking placebo. Other drug-related serious adverse events in the riociguat group included gastritis, acute renal failure, and hypotension.

■ Riociguat in Pregnancy

Riociguat is the first drug within its class of sGC stimulators. In an animal model, riociguat was consistently shown to have teratogenic effects when administered. It has been categorized as a Category X drug. If this drug is used during pregnancy or if the patient becomes pregnant while taking this drug, the patient should be informed of the potential hazard to the fetus. To prevent such situations, females of childbearing age should have testing for pregnancy before the start of treatment, monthly during treatment, and 1 month after stopping treatment. For all female patients, riociguat is available only through a restricted program called the Adempas REMS Program.

■ Drug Interactions

Riociguat is a direct stimulator of sGC leading to increased generation of cGMP which leads to vasodilatation. Riociguat is contraindicated when used with other drugs that increase cGMP availability. When co-administered with nitrates or NO donors (such as amyl nitrate), riociguat can cause a dramatic decrease in blood pressure and may lead to syncope.

The use of PDE inhibitors, especially PDE5 (sildenafil, tadalafil, and vardenafil) is also contraindicated with riociguat. These drugs are commonly used in PH. In one exploratory study, the addition of riociguat to a stable background therapy of sildenafil did not improve pulmonary hemodynamics, 6MWD, or WHO functional class compared to adding placebo but was associated with a higher rate of discontinuation due to hypotension.[12] Riociguat is also contraindicated with the use of nonspecific PDE inhibitors such as dipyridamole or theophylline.

Key Points

- Riociguat is the first of a new class of drugs that work by directly stimulating sGC activity and increasing sensitivity of sGC to NO.
- Riociguat is approved for the treatment of WHO Group 1 PAH and Group 4 CTEPH.
- Randomized trials of riociguat vs placebo have demonstrated improvement in 6MWD, pulmonary hemodynamics, and WHO functional class in patients with PAH or CTEPH.
- Riociguat is generally well tolerated. Major side effects include dizziness and headache.
- The use of riociguat is contraindicated in patients taking nitrates or PDE inhibitors or sexually active women of childbearing age who are not using a dual method of birth control.

9

REFERENCES

1. Ghofrani HA, Osterloh IH, Grimminger F. Sildenafil: from angina to erectile dysfunction to pulmonary hypertension and beyond. *Nat Rev Drug Discov*. 2006;5(8):689-702.

2. Evgenov OV, Pacher P, Schmidt PM, Haskó G, Schmidt HH, Stasch JP. NO-independent stimulators and activators of soluble guanylate cyclase: discovery and therapeutic potential. *Nat Rev Drug Discov*. 2006;5(9):755-768.

3. Grimminger F, Weimann G, Frey R, et al. First acute haemodynamic study of soluble guanylate cyclase stimulator riociguat in pulmonary hypertension. *Eur Respir J*. 2009;33(4):785-792.

4. Stasch JP, Hobbs AJ. NO-independent, haem-dependent soluble guanylate cyclase stimulators. *Handb Exp Pharmacol.* 2009;(191):277-308.

5. Mittendorf J, Weigand S, Alonso-Alija C, et al. Discovery of riociguat (BAY 63-2521): a potent, oral stimulator of soluble guanylate cyclase for the treatment of pulmonary hypertension. *ChemMedChem.* 2009;4(5):853-865.

6. Schermuly R, Stasch JP, Pullamsetti SS, et al. Expression and function of soluble guanylate cyclase in pulmonary arterial hypertension. *Eur Respir J.* 2008;32:881-891.

7. Ghofrani H-A, Hoeper MM, Halank M, et al. Riociguat for chronic thromboembolic pulmonary hypertension and pulmonary arterial hypertension: a phase II study. *Eur Respir J.* 2010;36:792-799.

8. Ghofrani HA, D'Armini AM, Grimminger F, et al. Riociguat for the treatment of chronic thromboembolic pulmonary hypertension. *N Engl J Med.* 2013;369(4):319-329.

9. Rubin LJ, Galiè N, Grimminger F, et al. Riociguat for the treatment of pulmonary arterial hypertension: a long-term extension study (PATENT-2) [published online ahead of print January 22, 2015]. *Eur Respir J.* doi: 10.1183/09031936.00090614.

10. Ghofrani HA, Galiè N, Grimminger F, et al. Riociguat for the treatment of pulmonary arterial hypertension. *N Engl J Med.* 2013;369(4):330-340.

11. Simonneau G, D'Armini AM, Ghofrani HA, et al. Riociguat for the treatment of chronic thromboembolic pulmonary hypertension: a long-term extension study (CHEST-2) [published online ahead of print November 13, 2014]. *Eur Respir J.* doi: 10/1183/09031936.00087114.

12. Galie N, Neuser D, Muller K Scalise A-V, Grunig E. A placebo-controlled, double-blind phase II interaction study to evaluate blood pressure following addition of riociguat to patients with symptomatic pulmonary arterial hypertension (PAH) receiving sildenafil (PATENT PLUS). *Am J Resp Crit Care Med.* 2013;187:A3530.

10

Adjunct Therapies and Supportive Care for PAH

by James R. Klinger, MD

Introduction

In addition to the four classes of medications that have been developed and approved specifically for the treatment of PAH, a variety of other therapies are commonly used to manage patients with this disease. These measures include medications such as diuretics, anticoagulants, and anti-arrhythmic drugs; supplemental oxygen; and cardiopulmonary rehabilitation. Although few of these therapies have been well studied, most address fairly obvious needs that arise during the treatment of chronic pulmonary vascular disease. Together, they have the potential to make important contributions to the care of patients with PAH while their affordability and ease of use provide little downside. As a result, the adjunct and supportive measures described below are often recommended on the basis of expert opinion and have been incorporated into recently published treatment guidelines.[1,2]

Diuretics

Diuretic therapy is the primary tool in the management of peripheral edema and volume overload in both left and right heart failure. Reducing preload by decreasing intravascular volume has been an effective method of reversing and preventing acute heart failure due to left ventricular systolic dysfunction. The same is likely to be true for the management of right heart failure associated with PAH. Although right ventricle systolic function is considerably more tolerant of increases in preload than the left ventricle, excessive intravascular volume can increase RV stroke work and elevated right-sided filling pressure (notably right atrial pressure) is a poor prognostic indicator in PAH.[3,4]

Determination of proper treatment goals for diuretic therapy in PAH can be challenging. As PAH progresses, the RV is subjected to an ever-increasing afterload that is partially compensated for by increased RV preload. At some point, however, further RV loading does little to enhance RV output and only increases RV volume leading to RV dilation and thinning of the RV free wall. As it enlarges, RV stroke work, which is proportional to RV chamber radius and inversely proportional to free wall thickness, can increase dramatically. The goal of diuretic therapy in PAH is to prevent overdistension of the RV, lessen RV stroke work, and improve cardiac output.

Correction of excessive right heart filling pressure can increase cardiac output and lead to substantial improvements in a patient's functional capacity and symptoms. Unfortunately, assessment of RV stroke work requires accurate measurement of RV pressure and output that usually requires invasive techniques. Thus, the practitioner must rely on clinical signs of RV failure such as elevated jugular venous distension and peripheral edema. In patients with RV failure from advanced PAH, it may not be possible to return these measures to normal, but every effort should be made to minimize them as much as possible. Echocardiography is useful for assessing the degree of RV enlargement and encroachment on LV filling[5] (**Figure 10.1**).

Movement of the interventricular septum toward the LV during diastole (often referred to as septal bowing or shift) suggests that RV end-diastolic pressure exceeds LV end-diastolic pressure and further reduction of RV preload is needed (**Figure 10.1**). Elevation of plasma BNP levels can also be an indicator of excess intravascular volume. At the same time, overaggressive use of diuretics can precipitate acute heart failure if RV filling pressures become too low.[6]

**FIGURE 10.1 — Ventricular Interdependence
in Pulmonary Hypertension**

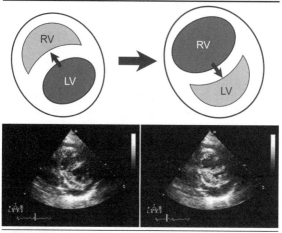

The position of the interventricular septum at end diastole is
determined by the difference between right and left ventricular end-diastolic pressure (RVEDP, LVEDP). Under normal
conditions, LVEDP is greater than RVEDP and the septum
bows toward the right ventricle during diastole. As the right
ventricle fails, RVEDP begins to exceed LVEDP and the
septum bows toward the left ventricle during diastole forming
a "D"-shaped pattern signaling RV pressure overload. When
right ventricular failure occurs due to elevated pulmonary
vascular resistance, increased intravascular volume raises
RVEDP further compromising left ventricular filling. Under
these circumstances, diuretic therapy can help reduce right
ventricular end-diastolic volume, thereby reducing RVEDP
and lessening the compromising effect of the right ventricle
on left ventricular filling.

Therefore, diuretic therapy must be individually titrated to minimize clinical signs of RV failure
without inducing a fall in cardiac output. In moderate cases of RV failure or volume overload, patients
can be followed closely as an outpatient with careful
laboratory monitoring of renal function and electrolyte
status. Potassium supplements are often required to
prevent hypokalemia, especially in patients on digoxin

therapy who may be at increased risk of developing cardiac arrhythmias. Salt and fluid restriction should be encouraged along with elevation of the legs whenever resting and the use of compressive stockings to control the accumulation of extracellular fluid in the lower extremities.

In severe RV failure, hospitalization may be required for monitoring of blood pressure, renal function, and electrolytes during diuretic therapy, particularly if a large volume of fluid is going to be removed quickly. Patients with chronically elevated right-sided filling pressures may have decreased absorbance of oral medications due to bowel wall edema and may require intravenous administration of diuretics.[6,7]

Anticoagulants

Histologic studies of lungs from PAH patients often reveal areas of pulmonary vascular thrombosis.[8,9] These lesions are not suggestive of systemic venous thrombi that have embolized to the lung but appear to have occurred in situ. A variety of abnormalities suggest that PAH is a prothrombotic disease. PAH is associated with a significant increase in the ratio of plasma thromboxane-to-prostacyclin levels.[10] Thromboxane is a major activator of thrombin and a potent vasoconstrictor, whereas prostacyclin is a potent endogenous inhibitor of platelet aggregation as well as a strong vasodilator. Thus, the increased thromboxane/prostacyclin ratio favors coagulation as well as vasoconstriction. Serotonin can facilitate platelet aggregation, and plasma levels are increased in PAH. Pulmonary vascular endothelial expression of abnormal von Willebrand factor has been reported in PAH and is associated with poorer short-term prognosis.[11] Abnormal levels of several other proteins involved in thrombosis and fibrinolysis have also been described in patients with PAH and may contribute to a hypercoagulable state.[12,13]

As a result of the increased risk of thrombosis, long-term anticoagulant therapy is felt to be an important part of the treatment of PAH. Unfortunately, this hypothesis has never been properly studied in randomized, placebo-controlled trials. There are, however, several open-label or retrospective studies that support the use of warfarin in the management of PAH. Three studies have retrospectively examined the association between anticoagulant use and survival.[7,14,15] All three found improved survival in those patients who were anticoagulated vs those who were not. Nearly all patients in the three studies had IPAH, HPAH, or PAH associated with anorectic drug use and were anticoagulated with warfarin.

The factors that determined whether or not a patient was anticoagulated were not identified. Thus, it is possible that the survival benefit was due to treatment bias (sicker patients may have had more difficulty being anticoagulated or less willing to be anticoagulated) rather than any effect of warfarin. However, in a recent study[16] that attempted to match disease severity between cases treated with and without anticoagulation, a survival advantage was still seen in IPAH patients treated with warfarin (**Figure 10.2**). The survival advantage was only seen in patients with IPAH and not in patients with PAH associated with scleroderma.

These results were consistent with an earlier study that found no effect of anticoagulation on outcome in PAH associated with scleroderma.[17] In the only prospective study of anticoagulants in PAH, patients treated with warfarin had about a 10% improvement in 5-year survival compared with patients who were not.[18] This uncontrolled, open-label study was designed to look at the efficacy of calcium channel blockers in patients with and without an acute pulmonary vasodilator response. The decision to use warfarin was determined by the presence of abnormal perfusion on lung perfusion (V/Q) scan and left to the discretion of the patient's physician. The improvement in survival was

FIGURE 10.2 — Effect of Anticoagulation on Survival of Patients With IPAH

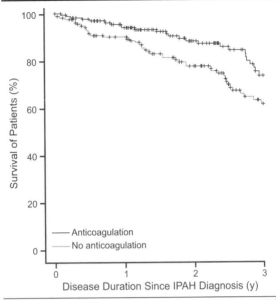

Effect of anticoagulation on survival of patients with idiopathic pulmonary arterial hypertension (IPAH) using a matched-pair analysis to control for disease severity. Survival was calculated from Kaplan-Mier estimates using 168 randomly matched pairs of patients based on sex, age, functional class, and pulmonary vascular resistance. The numbers of patients at risk at baseline and after 1, 2, and 3 years were 168, 124, 76, and 46, respectively, in the antico-agulation group and 168, 120, 84, and 41, respectively, in the no anticoagulation group.

Olsson KM, et al. *Circulation.* 2014;129(1):57-65.

seen in patients with and without a positive vasodilator response. The effect of anticoagulation on PAH associated with HIV infection, portopulmonary hypertension, or congenital heart disease has not been examined.

Whether the use of other anticoagulants such as the heparins, direct thrombin, or Factor Xa inhibitors improves outcomes in PAH is not known. In addition to its anticoagulant properties, unfractionated heparin blunts the development of PH in animal studies and in one study was more effective than warfarin at reversing hypoxia-induced PH in guinea pigs.[19] The effect of ASA has been studied in PAH but was found to be ineffective.[20] Current treatment guidelines for PAH recommend anticoagulation with a vitamin K+ antagonist and a targeted INR between 1.5 and 2.5 in patients with IPAH, HPAP, or PAH associated with anorexigens as long as the patient is not at an increased risk of bleeding.[2]

Supplemental Oxygen

Reduced oxygen tension in pulmonary circulation increases pulmonary vascular tone and can contribute to pulmonary vascular remodeling in a variety of ways. Hypoxia stimulates expression of a variety of growth factors implicated in the pathogenesis of PH such as HIF-1-alpha and can increase PVR by increasing blood viscosity from polycythemia. Exposure to chronic hypoxia has been shown to result in pulmonary vascular remodeling that is not completely reversible following return to normal oxygen tension. Care should be taken to make certain that reduced oxygen tension does not contribute to disease progression in patients with PAH. Although it may seem obvious that patients with PAH who are hypoxic on room air should benefit from supplemental oxygen, the effect of normalizing or raising oxygen saturation in PAH has not been formally studied.

Supplemental oxygen use for at least 15 hours a day led to small improvements in pulmonary hemodynamics in COPD patients enrolled in the Nocturnal Oxygen Therapy in Hypoxemic Chronic Obstructive Lung Disease Trial (NOTT).[21,22] However, the beneficial effect of oxygen in these COPD patients did not correlate with improvement in pulmonary hemodynamics. In fact, oxygen had a greater beneficial effect on survival in COPD patients with lower PVR than in those with higher PVR at baseline.[23]

Due to the lack of clinical studies in PAH, recommendations for the use of oxygen therapy in these patients are based on expert opinion. Considering the consistent effect of chronic hypoxia on inducing PH in numerous animal models as well as the high incidence of PH and right heart failure in human populations living at high altitude, it seems prudent that patients being treated for PAH be given supplemental oxygen as needed to prevent hypoxemia. The minimum level of hypoxia that is capable of causing PH in humans has not been determined, and individual pulmonary vasoconstrictive responses to hypoxia vary considerably. Thus, it is not clear what level of systemic arterial oxygen saturation should be maintained in patients with PAH. Current recommendations suggest the use of supplemental O_2 in PAH patients to maintain partial pressure of oxygen in arterial blood (PaO_2) >60 mm Hg.[2] In the United States, Medicare will reimburse the cost of supplemental oxygen for patients whose arterial oxygen saturation is <92% at rest on room air if there is evidence of PH.

An individual patient's acute pulmonary vasodilator response to oxygen can also be assessed during RHC. Occasionally, patients with low normal O_2 saturation may show improved pulmonary hemodynamics when their arterial O_2 saturation is increased. In these patients, it may be useful to maintain systemic arterial oxygen saturation at higher levels.

Patients should use their oxygen as often as possible, but for at least 18 hours a day and when sleeping. Patients with PAH who are normoxic at rest should be carefully assessed for intermittent hypoxia. Hypoxia associated with sleep disordered breathing or with exercise is common in patients with PAH.[24] Patients who only experience low oxygen saturation during sleep or exercise can limit their oxygen use to those periods.

Digoxin

The positive inotropic effects of digoxin and its beneficial effects in left heart failure have prompted some investigators to study its effect in right heart function in patients with PAH. Digoxin increases myocardial intracellular calcium concentrations by binding to the sodium-potassium ATPase and promoting sodium-calcium exchange. In healthy individuals, digoxin has little to no effect on cardiac output but has been shown to increase left ventricular ejection fraction in patients with congestive heart failure and reduce the incidence of hospitalizations and emergency room visits.

Limited data suggest that digoxin can improve RV function in patients with PAH, but the treatment effect is small and may not justify the potential adverse events. In one study,[25] cardiac output increased approximately 10% 2 hours after a single dose of digoxin in seventeen patients with PAH and right heart failure. A significant fall in norepinephrine levels and a trend toward a decrease in plasma renin activity was also seen. A similar improvement in RV function has also been demonstrated in PH associated with COPD, but in other studies of COPD patients, improvement in CO following 8 weeks of digoxin was limited to those who had reduced LV systolic function.[26] Due to the paucity of data showing benefit and its potential adverse arrhythmogenic effects, digoxin is not routinely recommended for the treatment of right heart failure in patients with PAH, although its use may be considered to slow ventricular rate in PAH patients with atrial tachyarrhythmias.[27]

Cardiopulmonary Rehabilitation

In its advanced stages, patients with PAH have considerable limitations of cardiovascular function and significant RV failure. Under these conditions, it would seem unwise to impose any additional cardiac load caused by stressful physical activity. Indeed, exercise-induced light-headedness or syncope is a clinical feature of advanced PAH. For these reasons, patients with PAH were often advised to refrain from stressful exercise. However, insufficient activity can lead to deconditioning and worsen cardiopulmonary function.

Over the last decade, several studies have examined the ability of specially designed exercise programs to improve cardiorespiratory function in patients with PAH. At least three randomized controlled trials have now shown that participation in a regular conditioning program improves functional capacity, including improvement in 6MWD (**Figure 10.3**) and quality of life in patients with PAH.[28] As a result, the most recently published WHO treatment guidelines recommend rehabilitation and exercise training for PAH patients and have upgraded this recommendation to its highest class and level of evidence.[2] These recommendations come with the understanding that the long-term effects of exercise training on survival and the best type and duration of exercise training are not known.

At a minimum, PAH patients participating in exercise programs should be monitored for oxygen saturation, symptoms, and blood pressure response during the design of their exercise program. It is recommended that patients participate in an exercise program that has experience with PAH patients and is in contact with a medical facility that specializes in diagnosis and treatment of PAH.[2]

Key Points

- In addition to PAH-specific medications, a variety of supportive measures including diuretics, anticoagulants, supplemental oxygen, and cardiopulmonary exercise training are frequently used in the management of PAH and are likely to be useful in selected patients.

FIGURE 10.3 — Effect of Exercise on 6MWD in Patients With PAH

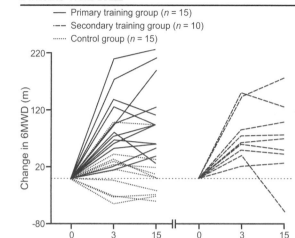

Mean (±SE) change in 6MWD from baseline to week 15 in the primary training, control, and secondary training groups (10 members of the control group reentered the study and received 15 weeks of exercise training).

$P=0.0003$ for primary training vs control group after 3 weeks of training. $P<0.0001$ for primary training vs control group after 15 weeks of training. $P<0.05$ for secondary training group vs control group after 3 weeks of training. $P=0.001$ for secondary training group vs control group after 15 weeks of training.

Mereles D, et al. *Circulation*. 2006;114:1482-1489.

10

- Patients with evidence of intravascular volume overload and right heart failure should be treated with diuretics while monitoring renal function and electrolyte imbalance.
- Care should be taken to assess for the presence of hypoxemia, including intermittent hypoxemia associated with sleep disordered breathing. Supplemental oxygen therapy should be considered in PAH patients who have a resting oxygen saturation <92%.

- Anticoagulation therapy should be considered for patients with idiopathic, heritable, or anorexigen-associated PAH who are not at increased risk of bleeding. Presently available evidence does not suggest a benefit of anticoagulation for patients with PAH associated with connective tissue disease.

REFERENCES

1. Taichman DB, Ornelas J, Chung L, et al. Pharmacologic therapy for pulmonary arterial hypertension in adults: CHEST guideline and expert panel report. *Chest*. 2014;146(2):449-475.

2. Galiè N, Corris PA, Frost A, et al. Updated treatment algorithm of pulmonary arterial hypertension. *J Am Coll Cardiol*. 2013;62(25 suppl):D60-D72.

3. D'Alonzo GE, Barst RJ, Ayres SM, et al. Survival in patients with primary pulmonary hypertension. Results from a national prospective registry. *Ann Int Med*. 1991;115:343-349.

4. Benza RL, Miller DP, Gomberg-Maitland M, et al. Predicting survival in pulmonary arterial hypertension: insights from the Registry to Evaluate Early and Long-Term Pulmonary Arterial Hypertension Disease Management (REVEAL). *Circulation*. 2010;122(2):164-172.

5. Gan CTJ, Lankhaar JWS, Marcus T, et al. Impaired left ventricular filling due to right-to-left ventricular interaction in patients with pulmonary arterial hypertension. *Am J Physiol Heart Circ Physiol*. 2006;290:H1528-H1533.

6. Alam S, Palevsky HI. Standard therapies for pulmonary arterial hypertension. *Clin Chest Med*. 2007;28:91-115.

7. Kawut SM, Horn EM, Berekashvili KK, et al. New predictors of outcomes in idiopathic pulmonary arterial hypertension. *Am J Cardiol*. 2005;95:199-203.

8. Bjornsson J, Edwards WD. Primary pulmonary hypertension: a histopathological study of 80 cases. *Mayo Clin Proc*. 1985;60:16-25.

9. Pietra GG, Edwards WD, Kay JM, et al. Histopathology of primary pulmonary hypertension. A qualitative and quantitative study of pulmonary vessels from 58 patients in the National Heart, Lung, and Blood Institute, Primary Pulmonary Hypertension Registry. *Circulation*. 1989;80:1198-1206.

10. Christman BW, McPherson CD, Newman JH, et al. An imbalance between the excretion of thromboxane and prostacyclin metabolites in pulmonary hypertension. *N Engl J Med*. 1992;327:70-75.

11. Lopes AA, Maeda NY. Circulating von Willebrand factor antigen as a predictor of short-term prognosis in pulmonary hypertension. *Chest*. 1998;114:1276-1282.

12. Can MM, Tanboga IH, Demircan HC, et al. Enhanced hemostatic indices in patients with pulmonary arterial hypertension: an observational study. *Thromb Res*. 2010;126:280-282.

13. Hoeper MM, Sosada M, Fabel H. Plasma coagulation profiles in patients with severe primary pulmonary hypertension. *Eur Resp J*. 1998;12:1446-1449.

14. Fuster V, Steele PM, Edwards WD, Gersh BJ, McGoon M, Frye RL. Primary pulmonary hypertension: natural history and importance of thrombosis. *Circulation*. 1984;70:580-587.

15. Frank H, Mlczoch J, Huber K, Schuster E, Gurtner HP, Kneussl M. The effect of anticoagulant therapy in primary and anorectic drug-induced pulmonary hypertension. *Chest*. 1997;112(3):714-721.

16. Olsson KM, Delcroix M, Ghofrani HA, et al. Anticoagulation and survival in pulmonary arterial hypertension: results from the Comparative, Prospective Registry of Newly Initiated Therapies for Pulmonary Hypertension (COMPERA). *Circulation*. 2014;129(1):57-65.

17. Johnson SR, Granton JT, Tomlinson GA, et al. Warfarin in systemic sclerosis-associated and idiopathic pulmonary arterial hypertension. A Bayesian approach to evaluation treatment for uncommon disease. *J Rheumatol*. 2012;39:276-285.

18. Rich S, Kaufman E, Levy PS. The effect of high doses of calcium-channel blockers on survival in primary pulmonary hypertension. *N Engl J Med*. 1992;327:76-81.

19. Hassoun PM, Thompson BT, Steigman D, Hales CA. Effect of heparin and warfarin on chronic hypoxic pulmonary hypertension and vascular remodeling in the guinea pig. *Am Rev Resp Dis*. 1989;139:763-768.

20. Robbins IM, Kawut SM, Yung D, et al. A study of aspirin and clopidogrel in idiopathic pulmonary hypertension. *Eur Resp J*. 2006;27:578-584.

21. Nocturnal Oxygen Therapy Trial Group. Continuous or nocturnal oxygen therapy in hypoxemic chronic obstructive lung disease. *Ann Int Med*. 1980;93:391-398.

10

22. Long term domiciliary oxygen therapy in chronic hypoxic corpulmonale complicating chronic bronchitis and emphysema: report of the Medical Research Council Working Party. *Lancet*. 1981;1:681-686.

23. Timms RM, Khaja FU, Williams GW;the Nocturnal Oxygen Therpay Trial Group. Hemodynamic response to oxygen therapy in chronic obstructive pulmonary disease. *Ann Int Med*. 1985;102:29-36.

24. Atwood CW, McCrory D, Garcia JG, Abman SH, Ahearn GS. Pulmonary artery hypertension and sleep-disordered breathing: ACCP evidence-based clinical practice guidelines. *Chest*. 2004;126:S72-S77.

25. Rich S, Seidlitz M, Dodin E, et al. The short-term effects of digoxin in patients with right ventricular dysfunction from pulmonary hypertension. *Chest*. 1998;114:787-792.

26. Mathur PN, Powles P, Pugsley SO, McEwan MP, Campell EJM. Effect of digoxin on right ventricular function in severe chronic airflow obstruction. *Ann Int Med*. 1981;95:283-288.

27. Galiè N, Hoeper M, Humbert M, et al. Guidelines on diagnosis and treatment of pulmonary hypertension: the Task Force on Diagnosis and Treatment of Pulmonary Hypertension of the European Society of Cardiology and of the European Respiratory Society. *Eur Heart J*. 2009;30:2493-2537.

28. Mereles D, Ehlken N, Kreuscher S, et al. Exercise and respiratory training improve exercise capacity and quality of life in patients with severe chronic pulmonary hypertension. *Circulation*. 2006;114:1482-1480.

11 Chronic Thromboembolic Pulmonary Hypertension

*by Arunabh Talwar, MD and
Sonu Sahni, MD*

Chronic thromboembolic pulmonary hypertension (CTEPH) or WHO Group 4 PH is defined by a mPAP >25 mm Hg in the presence of organized, nonacute thrombus within the pulmonary artery vascular bed.[1] CTEPH is the result of single or recurrent PE arising from sites of venous thrombosis. Distinguishing CTEPH from other forms of PH is of clinical importance because it carries significant morbidity and mortality and remains one of the few causes of PH that is surgically curable. Anatomic resolution of acute PE is not always complete. However, the great majority of patients who are properly treated will experience a return to normal pulmonary hemodynamics and functional status.[2] For reasons still unknown, a small subset of patients with a PE develop a pulmonary vascular hypertensive disease despite appropriate anticoagulation therapy.

Incidence

It is estimated that in the United States there are approximately 600,000 cases of PE of which 150,000 are diagnosed.[3] Analysis of registries suggests that the overall incidence of CTEPH is between 3 and 30 per 1 million in the general population.[4] The incidence of CTPEH after acute PE ranges from 0.6% to 8.8%.[5-8]

Miniati and colleagues reported that up to 35% of patients still have an abnormal ventilation-perfusion (V/Q) scan 1 year after their initial thromboembolic event.[7] In one prospective long-term follow-up study that assessed the incidence of symptomatic CTEPH in patients with an acute episode of PE, the cumulative incidence of symptomatic CTEPH was 1.0% (95% CI, 0.0-2.4) at 6 months, 3.1% (95% CI, 0.7-5.5) at 1 year, and 3.8% (95% CI, 1.1-6.5) at 2 years. No further cases of CTEPH were discovered after 2 years of follow-up in this cohort.[8] In another study, Klok and coworkers developed a cardiopulmonary screening program for CTEPH detection. They followed 866 unselected patients with acute PE for 34 months. The overall incidence of CTEPH was 0.57% (95% CI 0.02-1.2).[9]

Pathogenesis and Risk Factors

The current understanding of the pathogenesis of CTEPH is that there is a lack of resolution of acute PE that is due to either ineffective fibrinolysis and/or overactive inflammation and scarring of the acute clot. The result is the gradual formation of organized clot in the pulmonary artery vascular bed that becomes endothelialized and is no longer susceptible to thrombolysis.

The formation of pulmonary thromboembolism or in situ thrombosis may be instigated or aggravated by abnormalities in the clotting cascade, endothelial cells, or platelets, all of which interact in the coagulation process.[4] No abnormality of the coagulation or fibrinolytic pathway or of the pulmonary endothelium has been consistently identified, except for antiphospholipid antibody and elevated levels of factor VIII. The lupus anticoagulant is positive in approximately 10% of such patients, and 20% carry antiphospholipid antibodies, lupus anticoagulant, or both.[6] An acute PE that does not resolve completely is a risk factor for development of CTEPH, as is the presence of large perfusion defects on V/Q lung scan.[7,8,10] A diagram showing the various possible results of disturbed resolution of a thrombus is shown in **Figure 11.1**.

FIGURE 11.1 — Diagram Showing Various Possible Results of Disturbed Resolution of a Thrombus

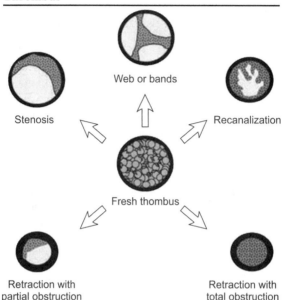

Castaner E, et al. *Radiographics*. 2009;29:31-53.

Clinical Presentation

The clinical presentation of CTEPH patients is similar to those of other causes of PH (**Table 11.1**). Patients who have a history of acute PE may report never recovering to their normal level of breathing or having a period of time where they are asymptomatic with exertional symptoms appearing months or years after the initial event. However, approximately 30% to 40% of CTEPH patients report no prior history of thromboembolic disease, making it necessary to consider CTEPH in all cases of PH without a known etiology.[12] Exertional dyspnea and exercise intolerance are the most common complaints and are thought to

TABLE 11.1 — Is There a Reason to Suspect PAH?

Not a PAH subgroup, but...
- Should never be missed
- Is potentially curable with thromboendarterectomy
- 3% to 4% of acute PE do not entirely resolve
- Only half of those with CTEPH have a history of acute PE
- Normal V/Q scan excludes chronic PE

McLaughlin VV, et al. *J Am Coll Cardiol.* 2009;53:1573-1619.

occur because of increased dead space ventilation.[11] In addition to exertional symptoms, unexplained dyspnea, dizziness, near-syncope, true syncope, and exertional chest pain are all possible signs and symptoms in these patients.[11]

In early disease, physical examination may be normal or limited to a subtle prominence of the pulmonic component of the second heart sound. However, as the disease progresses, the findings on physical examination are similar to other PH patients. Patients may exhibit increased jugular venous pressure, a loud or split second heart sound with an increased P2 component, a tricuspid regurgitation murmur, a right ventricular (RV) heave, or a RV S4 gallop.[13] The murmur of the tricuspid valve is likely secondary to a dilated tricuspid annulus in the setting of RV volume and pressure overload. Often this murmur improves or resolves completely after thromboendarterectomy if the PASP is <40 mm Hg postoperatively.

Another physical finding which is now rarely described in the literature is pulmonary flow murmurs. Auger and colleagues reported that approximately 30% of patients have a pulmonary flow murmur, a bruit caused by turbulent blood flow through pulmonary arteries partially obstructed by chronic thrombus.[14,15] Presence of this murmur is a pathognomonic sign for CTEPH and should warrant further investigation. In addition, as CTEPH progresses, there is augmentation of right heart failure and patients may develop hepatomegaly, ascites, and lower extremity edema.

Diagnosis and Evaluation

In patients with suspected CTEPH, the primary objective is to confirm the actual presence of thromboembolic pulmonary vascular obstruction and to assess the extent of hemodynamic impairment.[1] Once the diagnosis of CTEPH is established, a subsequent management decision exists based on certain factors such as the quantity and accessibility of clot, and an estimation of the anticipated postoperative hemodynamic result. Suspicion of CTEPH should be high whenever a patient presents with PH and a previous history of venous thromboembolism.

■ Workup

Chest X-Ray

A chest radiograph may be normal in the early stages of the disease. In advanced CTEPH, Woodruff and associates found that signs frequently found in CTEPH were cardiomegaly (86%), oligemia (68%), right descending pulmonary artery enlargement (55%), effusion (23%), and pleural thickening (14%).[16] Other signs often seen in PE patients, who make up the majority of patients who develop CTEPH, include clear lung fields with areas of hypoperfusion (Westermark sign) or evidence of previous infarction (Hampton hump). In one study, the presence of oligemia was pathognomonic for CTEPH.[17]

Pulmonary Function Testing

Patients without coexisting pulmonary pathologies typically have normal spirometry and lung volumes, although some have shown a restrictive ventilatory defect.[18] The D_{LCO} may be may be normal, mildly reduced, or moderately reduced.[19] Severe reductions in D_{LCO} should prompt consideration of underlying parenchymal abnormalities such as interstitial lung disease.

Transthoracic Echocardiography (TTE)

TTE is an effective method of screening for PH in patients who are suspected of having CTEPH. Pulmonary artery systolic pressure can be estimated using a Doppler analysis of the tricuspid regurgitant jet, and right heart size and systolic function can be assessed.[20,21] If PH is detected on TTE, right heart catheterization is needed to confirm the presence of elevated PAP and assess its severity and rule out other etiologies such as elevated pulmonary venous pressure.

Ventilation-Perfusion Scanning (V/Q Scanning)

V/Q scanning remains the test of choice to rule out CTEPH. A completely normal perfusion study essentially excludes the diagnosis of surgically accessible CTEPH.[22-24] V/Q scanning is important because it can distinguish CTEPH patients from those with PAH.[21,25,26] Patients with CTEPH show one or more segmental or larger unmatched perfusion defects. On the other hand, patients with PAH have normal or mottled perfusion scans with subsegmental perfusion defects.[23,24] V/Q scanning is more sensitive than multidetector CT pulmonary angiography.[27] However, V/Q scanning does not anatomically localize the extent of disease nor does it indicate surgical accessibility which can be better established by CT pulmonary angiography (**Figure 11.2**).

Computer Tomography Pulmonary Angiography (CTPA)

Although not an ideal screening tool for CTEPH, CT angiography is very useful and sensitive in the evaluation of CTEPH with more central and segmental disease burden. In a small study of 27 patients with CTEPH, 64-detector row CT scan had a diagnostic sensitivity of 98.3% at the main and lobar level and 94% at the segmental level.[28] In addition to imaging the pulmonary vasculature, CTPA may provide important information about the rest of the lung such as parenchyma and pleura.

FIGURE 11.2 — Ventilation-Perfusion Scan Showing Filling Defects in Both Right and Left Lobes

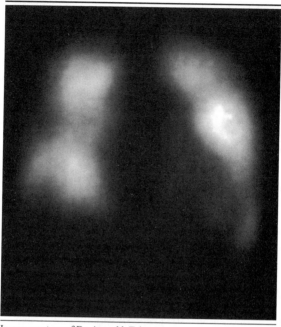

Image courtesy of Dr. Arunabh Talwar.

Chronic thromboemboli appear as complete or partial vascular obstructions, eccentric filling defects, intraluminal webs, or bands. The lung parenchyma often shows mosaic attenuation of perfusion[29,30] (see *Chapter 4*). In comparison to conventional pulmonary angiography, detection rates for central emboli with CTPA were similar in 55 patients suspected of having CTEPH, although detection of segmental disease was superior with conventional pulmonary angiography.[29] In addition, CT scanning provides additional valuable information in the evaluation of CTEPH, including:

- Presence and extent of parenchymal disease;
- Anatomy and size of pulmonary arteries and vessels;

- Location of arterial webs and bands; and
- Location of collateral vessels in the mediastinum.[31]

Figure 11.3 shows a CT scan with chronic thrombus in segments of the right pulmonary artery.

FIGURE 11.3 — CT Scan Showing Chronic Thrombus in Segments of Right Pulmonary Artery

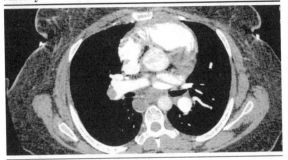

Image courtesy of Dr. Arunabh Talwar.

MRI of Pulmonary Vessels

The role of MRI has been increasing, not only in the detection of chronic thromboembolic disease but also in the assessment of right ventricular function and its response to therapy. With experienced clinicians, magnetic resonance angiography has been shown to accurately show findings of CTEPH (intraluminal webs/bands, vessel cutoffs, and organized central thromboemboli) up to the segmental level.[32,33] In addition, three-dimensional contrast-enhanced lung perfusion MRI tracks the dynamic passage of a contrast bolus, allowing imaging of regional pulmonary perfusion. A recent study investigated 132 patients with PH, all of whom underwent perfusion scintigraphy, lung perfusion MRI, CTPA, and right heart catheterization at a large PH referral center. Seventy-eight patients were confirmed to have CTEPH. Sensitivity in the diagnosis of CTEPH was 96% for perfusion scintigraphy, 97%

for MR perfusion, and 94% for CTPA.[34] Disadvantages include the usual contraindications to MRI such as claustrophobia, pacemakers, and foreign metallic objects.

Conventional Pulmonary Angiography

Pulmonary angiography remains the gold standard for diagnosis of CTEPH. It also helps in decision-making of surgical intervention. Characteristic features in CTEPH include vascular webs, intimal irregularities, intraluminal defects, and abrupt narrowing of vessels.

Right Heart Catheterization

Despite the availability of multiple imaging techniques to help determine the presence of chronic emboli, RHC is necessary for diagnosis of CTEPH. The severity of PH cannot be predicted by the degree of clot burden and TTE can significantly over- or under-estimate pulmonary pressure. In addition to confirming the presence of elevated pulmonary pressure, RHC provides important information regarding the severity of PH that is present, right and left heart filling pressures, and cardiac output. This information is important for excluding other causes of PH such as left-sided heart disease and determining whether pulmonary endarterectomy is indicated. In some institutions, RHC may be performed at the time of pulmonary angiography.

11

Treatment

■ Surgery

The only curative option for patients with CTEPH is surgical removal of thromboembolic material and obstructive lesions within the pulmonary arteries by a procedure known as pulmonary endarterectomy (PEA).[21,35] This well-described procedure has the following goals when treating CTEPH[36,37]:

- *Hemodynamic*: to improve RV function by reducing the PVR and PAP
- *Respiratory*: to restore perfusion to the large areas of ventilation

- *Prophylactic*: to prevent further deterioration in RV function and progressive, secondary arteriopathic changes in the pulmonary vasculature.

Due to improved surgical techniques, PEA has become the gold standard for treatment of CTEPH, resulting in a significant reduction of PAP and improvement in RV function, quality of life, and survival.[21,35] Preoperative eligibility criteria for CTEPH varies between centers; however, clinical guidelines provided by the American College of Chest Physicians are widely used and provide a basic framework to assess the operability of patients with CTEPH[39] (**Table 11.2**).

TABLE 11.2 — Eligibility Criteria for PEA

- NYHA function class III or IV symptoms
- Preoperative PVR >300 dyn·sec·cm^{-5}
- Mean PAP >40 mm Hg
- Surgically accessible thrombus in the main, lobar, or segmental pulmonary arteries
- No severe medical comorbidities
- Absence of secondary arteriopathy
- Predicted reduction of PVR of >50%
- Center experience
- Patient consent

Doyle RL, et al. *Chest*. 2004;126(1 suppl):63S-71S.

Perioperative assessment is made regarding the classification of thrombus, and the most widely used scheme has been proposed by Thistlewaite and colleagues (**Table 11.3**).[36] Type 1 and 2 disease is more surgically accessible and has better outcomes, while Type 3 and 4 disease is associated with an increased perioperative mortality and greater postoperative PVR.[36] Surgical outcome measures typically reported include in-hospital mortality, reduction in PAP and PVR, and improvement in NYHA heart failure classification, 6MWD, and long-term survival. A marked reduction in mPAP and an improvement in cardiac output is often seen immediately following PEA.[41]

TABLE 11.3 — Classification of CTEPH

Type	Description
1	Fresh thrombus within the main and/or lobar-pulmonary arteries
2	Intimal thickening and fibrosis proximal to the segmental arteries
3	Disease within the distal segmental arteries only
4	Distal arterial vasculopathy with no visible thromboembolic material

Thistlethwaite PA, et al. J *Thorac Cardiovasc Surg.* 2002;124(6): 1203-1211.

Operative mortality rates after PEA range from 4% to 30% depending on center experience, patient selection, and comorbidities,[37,38,42] but most centers report successful surgery and 1-year survival in excess of 95%.[37,38] International registry data report that within 1 year after surgery, the median PVR decreased from 698 to 235 dyn·sec·cm^{-5} and the median 6MWD increased from 362 to 459 m.[38]

General predictors of successful outcomes from PEA have been outlined as[35]:

- Prior history of PE and/or deep venous thrombosis
- A honeymoon period of months to years between the embolic event and clinical development of CTEPH
- Appropriate association between anatomic lesions and PH/PVR
- Angiographic lesions located in the proximal PA and lobar branches.

Some patients may not achieve normal pulmonary pressures or right heart function after thromboendarectomy. Preoperative indicators of postoperative complications include increased PVR, >1000 dyn·sec·cm^{-5}. Madani and colleagues reported a mortality of 10% in those patients who had a PVR of >500 dyn·sec·cm^{-5} postoperatively compared with 0.9% when postoperative PVR was <500 dyn·sec·cm^{-5}.[41] PEA is a difficult surgery that requires extensive cardiopulmonary bypass and temporary cardiac arrest and may be too demanding for some patients to endure. However, the immediate and long-term results are usually significantly better than medical therapy and patients should be given every opportunity to undergo this procedure. Patients with CTEPH should be evaluated by a center that is well experienced in the diagnosis and surgical treatment of CTEPH before they are deemed to be a nonsurgical candidate. Many patients who have what appears to be a relatively small proximal clot burden may be found to have more extensive disease with partially recannulized lesions or webs in the first or second order pulmonary arteries that can benefit from surgical resection.

In patients where PEA is not an option, bilateral lung transplantation may be considered. Due to lack donors, lung transplantation is rare in CTEPH patients. Results of lung transplantation for CTEPH show a 1-year survival of 80% and 5-year survival ranging from 52% to 60%. In addition, the need for lifelong immunosuppression is coupled with risk of increased infection.[40]

■ Medical Therapy

Medical therapy in CTEPH has been reserved for:
- Patients deemed to have inoperable CTEPH
- Patients with residual PH after PEA
- A therapeutic bridge in those patients with operable chronic thromboembolic disease with severe PH and right heart dysfunction.

Lifelong anticoagulation therapy is prescribed for most patients with CTEPH to prevent in situ pulmonary artery thrombosis and the recurrence of acute PE. In addition, some patients with CTEPH may also benefit from selective pulmonary vasodilator therapy. Over the past decade, many medications have been developed for the treatment of PAH and most have been used for the treatment of CTEPH as well. These medications include prostanoids, endothelin receptor blockers, phosphodiesterase-5 inhibitors, and, most recently, the soluble guanylate cyclase stimulator riociguat. At present, riociguat is the only drug approved by the FDA for the treatment of CTEPH (see *Chapter 9*).

Riociguat

Riociguat is a direct sGC stimulator that was recently approved by the FDA for the treatment of PAH and CTEPH. It is indicated for the treatment of adults with persistent/recurrent CTEPH after surgical treatment or inoperable CTEPH. Riociguat helps patients improve exercise capacity and degree of symptoms indicated by the WHO functional class.

The efficacy and safety of riociguat was examined in a randomized, double-blind, placebo-controlled trial in patients with inoperable or recurrent/persistent CTEPH (CHEST-1).[43] In CHEST-1, riociguat was found to significantly improve exercise capacity and PVR compared with placebo in patients with CTEPH. See *Chapter 9* for a more detailed description of the CHEST-1 trial.

Prostacyclin Analogues

Prostacyclin is an endogenous substance produced by vascular endothelial cells and induces vasodilatation and inhibition of platelet activity, and has possible antiproliferative effects.[44] The use of prostacyclins to treat CTEPH is based on the role of prostacyclin in vasculopathy and the PAH disease process. Prostanoids have been shown to reduce PVR and improve RV function. Together with evidence of efficacy from clinical trials in PAH, this provides a rationale for their possible application in CTEPH.

The use of intravenous epoprostenol, a prostacyclin derivative, in patients with inoperable CTEPH has also been examined. In a recent study specifically addressing this issue, Cabrol and colleagues[45] retrospectively analyzed 27 patients with inoperable CTEPH who were treated with epoprostenol. After 3 months of therapy, there was a decrease in mPAP (56 ± 9 mm Hg to 51 ± 8 mm Hg), total pulmonary resistance (29.3 ± 7.0 U/m^2 to 23.0 ± 5.0 U/m^2), and an increase in 6MWD of 66 m. NYHA functional class improved by one tier in 11 of 23 patients.[45]

In a single-center uncontrolled observational study,[46] 28 patients with severe inoperable CTEPH were treated with subcutaneous treprostinil (a prostacyclin analogue). Right heart catheterization was repeated in 19 patients after 19 ± 6.3 months of treatment. Treprostinil therapy was associated not only with a significant reduction in PVR but also an improvement 6MWD, WHO functional class, brain natriuretic peptide (BNP) levels, and CO. Five-year survival rate was 53% compared with 16% in untreated historical controls.[46]

There are limited data on inhaled iloprost in patients with inoperable CTEPH. In a study of 20 patients with CTEPH (12 with distal chronic thromboembolic lesions), with an administration of 5 µg of iloprost, Krug and colleagues showed an acute hemodynamic response with a slight decline in PVR and mPAP with an increase in CO.[47] Acknowledging that 16 of the 20 patients were already receiving one or more PAH-specific medical therapies at the time, the investigators' observation of an acute hemodynamic response to inhaled iloprost suggested there might be a component of vasoconstriction in this subgroup of patients with CTEPH. This finding supports a similar observation made by Ulrich and colleagues in which acute vasoreactivity to 10 µg of inhaled iloprost was shown in 22 patients with CTEPH.[48]

Endothelin Receptor Antagonists (ERAs)

Bosentan is the ERA that has been studied the most in CTEPH. In a meta-analysis involving 11 studies comprising 269 patients (39 patients with persistent PH following endarterectomy), treatment with bosentan was associated with an improvement in 6MWD of 35.9 m after 3 to 6 months of therapy. Approximately 25% of patients experienced an improvement in NYHA functional class during this same follow-up period. An additional gain of 21 m at 1 year was achieved for patients receiving drug for a more extended period. Hemodynamic data available from seven studies (185 patients) revealed a weighted improvement in cardiac index (0.23 L/min/m^2), reduction in mPAP (2.62 mm Hg), and, in five studies (164 patients), a reported weighted mean reduction in PVR of 159.7 dyn·sec·cm^{-5} (20% of baseline).[49]

The only randomized controlled trial examining the efficacy of bosentan in inoperable CTEPH was reported in 2008. Jais and colleagues[53] enrolled 157 patients (bosentan use in 77 patients) with approximately 28% having previously undergone PTE surgery. Compared with baseline, 16-week treatment with bosentan resulted in an improvement in pulmonary hemodynamic parameters: a 24.1% reduction in PVR and a decline in total pulmonary resistance (treatment effect, -193 dyn·sec·cm^{-5}) with an increase in cardiac index (treatment effect, 0.3 L/min/m^2). There was also a decrease in NT-proBNP levels (-622 ng/L) in the bosentan-treated patients relative to those receiving placebo. However, at 16 weeks, there was no definable improvement in exercise capacity (6MWD) and no statistically significant treatment effect of bosentan on WHO functional class.[50]

Phosphodiesterase-5 Inhibitors

PDE5 inhibitors have been studied for CTEPH in clinical trials. In a double-blind, placebo-controlled, 12-week pilot study, Suntharalingham and colleagues[51] enrolled 19 patients with inoperable CTEPH, assessing the benefit of sildenafil (nine patients receiving drug) in this group. There was no significant difference detected in 6MWD (primary endpoint). However, an improvement in WHO functional class and PVR were noted. Control subjects were then transitioned to open-label sildenafil use and reassessed at 12 months. Significant improvement in 6MWD, activity, and symptom scores (as measured on the Cambridge Pulmonary Hypertension Outcome Review [CAMPHOR] Quality of Life questionnaire), cardiac index, PVR, and NT-proBNP values (1000-811 pg/ mL) were noted.

11

In a larger patient group, Reichenberger and colleagues[52] conducted an open-label study of sildenafil (50 mg 3 times a day) in 104 patients with inoperable CTEPH. After 3 months of therapy, there was a modest decrease in PVR (863 ± 38 dyn·sec·cm^{-5} to 759 ± 62 dyn·sec·cm^{-5}), with an increase in 6MWD from 310 ± 11 m to 361 ± 15 m; this distance further improved to 366 ± 18 m after 12 months of sildenafil.[52]

Key Points

- CTEPH or WHO Group 4 PH is defined by a mPAP >25 mm Hg in the presence of organized, nonacute thrombus within the pulmonary artery vascular bed.

- Clinical presentation of CTEPH patients is similar to those of other causes of PH. Patients who have a history of PE may report a period of time where they are asymptomatic after the event with exertional dyspnea appearing months or years after the initial event.

- The diagnostic evaluation of CTEPH serves to confirm obstructing chronic thromboembolic disease as the cause of PH and quantify its hemodynamic impact, to determine the surgical accessibility of the disease, to estimate the likelihood of symptomatic and hemodynamic benefit from surgical resection, and to assess comorbidities that may affect perioperative short-term and long-term outcomes of PEA surgery.

- The diagnostic workup of CTEPH usually requires a V/Q scan, which is the most sensitive screening test, and CT or conventional pulmonary angiography to determine the amount and accessibility of clot for surgical resection.

- Surgical eligibility should be determined by centers that are well experienced in the diagnosis and surgical treatment of CTEPH.

- Patients who appropriate surgical candidates should be offered PEA.

- Patients who are poor surgical candidates or who do not have surgically accessible clot should be treated with the soluble guanylate cyclase stimulator riociguat (see *Chapter 9*).
- Riociguat should also be considered in patients who have symptomatic PH following PEA.

11

REFERENCES

1. Marshall PS, Kerr KM, Auger WR. Chronic thromboembolic pulmonary hypertension. *Clin Chest Med*. 2013;34(4):779-797.

2. Fedullo P, Kerr KM, Kim NH, Auger WR. Chronic thromboembolic pulmonary hypertension. *Am J Respir Crit Care Med*. 2011;183(12):1605-1613.

3. Kucher N, Goldhaber SZ. Management of massive pulmonary embolism. *Circulation*. 2005;112(2):e28-e32.

4. Lang IM, Pesavento R, Bonderman D, Yuan JX. Risk factors and basic mechanisms of chronic thromboembolic pulmonary hypertension: a current understanding. *Eur Respir J*. 2013;41(2):462-468.

5. Becattini C, Agnelli G, Pesavento R, et al. Incidence of chronic thromboembolic pulmonary hypertension after a first episode of pulmonary embolism. *Chest*. 2006;130(1):172-175.

6. Dentali F, Donadini M, Gianni M, et al. Incidence of chronic pulmonary hypertension in patients with previous pulmonary embolism. *Thromb Res*. 2009;124(3):256-258.

7. Miniati M, Monti S, Bottai M, et al. Survival and restoration of pulmonary perfusion in a long-term follow-up of patients after acute pulmonary embolism. *Medicine (Baltimore)*. 2006;85(5):253-262.

8. Pengo V, Lensing AW, Prins MH, et al; Thromboembolic Pulmonary Hypertension Study Group. Incidence of chronic thromboembolic pulmonary hypertension after pulmonary embolism. *N Engl J Med*. 2004;350(22):2257-2264.

9. Klok FA, van Kralingen KW, van Dijk AP, Heyning FH, Vliegen HW, Huisman MV. Prospective cardiopulmonary screening program to detect chronic thromboembolic pulmonary hypertension in patients after acute pulmonary embolism. *Haematologica*. 2010;95(6):970-975.

10. Piazza G, Goldhaber SZ. Chronic thromboembolic pulmonary hypertension. *N Engl J Med*. 2011;364(4):351-360.

11. Kapitan KS, Buchbinder M, Wagner PD, Moser KM. Mechanisms of hypoxemia in chronic thromboembolic pulmonary hypertension. *Am Rev Respir Dis*. 1989;139(5):1149-1154.

12. Pepke-Zaba J, Delcroix M, Lang I, et al. Chronic thromboembolic pulmonary hypertension (CTEPH): results from an international prospective registry. *Circulation*. 2011;124(18):1973-1981.

13. Haythe J. Chronic thromboembolic pulmonary hypertension: a review of current practice. *Prog Cardiovasc Dis.* 2012;55(2):134-143.

14. ZuWallack RL, Liss JP, Lahiri B. Acquired continuous murmur associated with acute pulmonary thromboembolism. *Chest.* 1976;70(4):557-559.

15. Auger WR, Moser KM. Pulmonary flow murmurs: a distinctive physical sign found in chronic pulmonary thromboembolic disease. *Clin Res.* 1989;37:145A.

16. Woodruff WW 3rd, Hoeck BE, Chitwood WR Jr, Lyerly HK, Sabiston DC Jr, Chen JT. Radiographic findings in pulmonary hypertension from unresolved embolism. *AJR Am J Roentgenol.* 1985;144(4):681-686.

17. Anderson GJ, Woodburn R, Fisch C. Cerebrovascular accident with unusual ectrocardiographic changes. *Am Heart J.* 1973;86(3):395-398.

18. Morris TA, Auger WR, Ysrael MZ, et al. Parenchymal scarring is associated with restrictive spirometric defects in patients with chronic thromboembolic pulmonary hypertension. *Chest.* 1996;110(2):399-403.

19. Bernstein RJ, Ford RL, Clausen JL, Moser KM. Membrane diffusion and capillary blood volume in chronic thromboembolic pulmonary hypertension. *Chest.* 1996;110(6):1430-1436.

20. Dittrich HC, McCann HA, Blanchard DG. Cardiac structure and function in chronic thromboembolic pulmonary hypertension. *Am J Card Imaging.* 1994;8(1):18-27.

21. Galiè N, Hoeper MM, Humbert M, et al; ESC Committee for Practice Guidelines (CPG). Guidelines for the diagnosis and treatment of pulmonary hypertension: the Task Force for the Diagnosis and Treatment of Pulmonary Hypertension of the European Society of Cardiology (ESC) and the European Respiratory Society (ERS), endorsed by the International Society of Heart and Lung Transplantation (ISHLT). *Eur Heart J.* 2009;30(20):2493-2537.

22. Fishman AJ, Moser KM, Fedullo PF. Perfusion lung scans vs pulmonary angiography in evaluation of suspected primary pulmonary hypertension. *Chest.* 1983;84(6):679-683.

23. Lisbona R, Kreisman H, Novales-Diaz J, Derbekyan V. Perfusion lung scanning: differentiation of primary from thromboembolic pulmonary hypertension. *AJR Am J Roentgenol.* 1985;144(1):27-30.

24. Powe JE, Palevsky HI, McCarthy KE, Alavi A. Pulmonary arterial hypertension: value of perfusion scintigraphy. *Radiology.* 1987;164(3):727-730.

11

25. Wilkens H, Lang I, Behr J, et al. Chronic thromboembolic pulmonary hypertension (CTEPH): updated Recommendations of the Cologne Consensus Conference 2011. *Int J Cardiol.* 2011;154 Suppl 1:S54-S60.

26. McLaughlin VV, Archer SL, Badesch DB, et al; ACCF/AHA. ACCF/AHA 2009 expert consensus document on pulmonary hypertension: a report of the American College of Cardiology Foundation Task Force on Expert Consensus Documents and the American Heart Association: developed in collaboration with the American College of Chest Physicians, American Thoracic Society, Inc., and the Pulmonary Hypertension Association. *Circulation.* 2009;119(16):2250-2294.

27. Tunariu N, Gibbs SJ, Win Z, et al. Ventilation-perfusion scintigraphy is more sensitive than multidetector CTPA in detecting chronic thromboembolic pulmonary disease as a treatable cause of pulmonary hypertension. *J Nucl Med.* 2007;48(5):680-684.

28. Reichelt A, Hoeper MM, Galanski M, Keberle M. Chronic thromboembolic pulmonary hypertension: evaluation with 64-detector row CT versus digital substraction angiography. *Eur J Radiol.* 2009;71(1):49-54.

29. Bergin CJ, Sirlin CB, Hauschildt JP, et al. Chronic thromboembolism: diagnosis with helical CT and MR imaging with angiographic and surgical correlation. *Radiology.* 1997;204(3):695-702.

30. Willemink MJ, van Es HW, Koobs L, Morshuis WJ, Snijder RJ, van Heesewijk JP. CT evaluation of chronic thromboembolic pulmonary hypertension. *Clin Radiol.* 2012;67(3):277-285.

31. Castañer E, Gallardo X, Ballesteros E, et al. CT diagnosis of chronic pulmonary thromboembolism. *Radiographics.* 2009;29(1):31-50; discussion 50-53.

32. Kovacs G, Reiter G, Reiter U, Rienmüller R, Peacock A, Olschewski H. The emerging role of magnetic resonance imaging in the diagnosis and management of pulmonary hypertension. *Respiration.* 2008;76(4):458-470.

33. Kreitner KF, Ley S, Kauczor HU, et al. Chronic thromboembolic pulmonary hypertension: pre- and postoperative assessment with breath-hold MR imaging techniques. *Radiology.* 2004;232(2):535-543.

34. Rajaram S, Swift AJ, Telfer A, et al. 3D contrast-enhanced lung perfusion MRI is an effective screening tool for chronic thromboembolic pulmonary hypertension: results from the ASPIRE Registry. *Thorax.* 2013;68(7):677-678.

35. Klepetko W, Mayer E, Sandoval J, et al. Interventional and surgical modalities of treatment for pulmonary arterial hypertension. *J Am Coll Cardiol*. 2004;43(12 Suppl S):73S-80S.

36. Thistlethwaite PA, Mo M, Madani MM, et al. Operative classification of thromboembolic disease determines outcome after pulmonary endarterectomy. *J Thorac Cardiovasc Surg*. 2002;124(6):1203-1211.

37. Jamieson SW, Kapelanski DP, Sakakibara N, et al. Pulmonary endarterectomy: experience and lessons learned in 1,500 cases. *Ann Thorac Surg*. 2003;76(5):1457-1462; discussion 1462-1464.

38. Mayer E, Jenkins D, Lindner J, et al. Surgical management and outcome of patients with chronic thromboembolic pulmonary hypertension: results from an international prospective registry. *J Thorac Cardiovasc Surg*. 2011;141(3):702-710.

39. Doyle RL, McCrory D, Channick RN, Simonneau G, Conte J; American College of Chest Physicians. Surgical treatments/interventions for pulmonary arterial hypertension: ACCP evidence-based clinical practice guidelines. *Chest*. 2004;126(1 Suppl):63S-71S.

40. Fadel E, Mercier O, Mussot S, et al. Long-term outcome of double-lung and heart-lung transplantation for pulmonary hypertension: a comparative retrospective study of 219 patients. *Eur J Cardiothorac Surg*. 2010;38(3):277-284.

41. Madani MM, Auger WR, Pretorius V, et al. Pulmonary endarterectomy: recent changes in a single institution's experience of more than 2,700 patients. *Ann Thorac Surg*. 2012;94(1):97-103; discussion 103.

42. Freed DH, Thomson BM, Tsui SS, et al. Functional and haemodynamic outcome 1 year after pulmonary thromboendarterectomy. *Eur J Cardiothorac Surg*. 2008;34(3):525-529; discussion 529-530.

43. Ghofrani HA, D'Armini AM, Grimminger F et al; CHEST-1 Study Group. Riociguat for the treatment of chronic thromboembolic pulmonary hypertension. *N Engl J Med*. 2013;369(4):319-329.

44. Galiè N, Manes A, Branzi A. Prostanoids for pulmonary arterial hypertension. *Am J Respir Med*. 2003;2(2):123-137.

45. Cabrol S, Souza R, Jais X, et al. Intravenous epoprostenol in inoperable chronic thromboembolic pulmonary hypertension. *J Heart Lung Transplant*. 2007;26(4):357-362.

46. Skoro-Sajer N, Bonderman D, Wiesbauer F, et al. Treprostinil for severe inoperable chronic thromboembolic pulmonary hypertension. *J Thromb Haemost*. 2007;5(3):483-489.

11

47. Krug S, Hammerschmidt S, Pankau H, Wirtz H, Seyfarth HJ. Acute improved hemodynamics following inhaled iloprost in chronic thromboembolic pulmonary hypertension. *Respiration*. 2008;76(2):154-159.

48. Ulrich S, Fischler M, Speich R, Popov V, Maggiorini M. Chronic thromboembolic and pulmonary arterial hypertension share acute vasoreactivity properties. *Chest*. 2006;130(3):841-846.

49. Becattini C, Manina G, Busti C, Gennarini S, Agnelli G. Bosentan for chronic thromboembolic pulmonary hypertension: findings from a systematic review and meta-analysis. *Thromb Res*. 2010;126(1):e51-e56.

50. Jaïs X, D'Armini AM, Jansa P, et al; Bosentan Effects in iNopErable Forms of chronIc Thromboembolic pulmonary hypertension Study Group. Bosentan for treatment of inoperable chronic thromboembolic pulmonary hypertension: BENEFiT (Bosentan Effects in iNopErable Forms of chronIc Thromboembolic pulmonary hypertension), a randomized, placebo-controlled trial. *J Am Coll Cardiol*. 2008;52(25):2127-2134.

51. Suntharalingam J, Treacy CM, Doughty NJ, et al. Long-term use of sildenafil in inoperable chronic thromboembolic pulmonary hypertension. *Chest*. 2008;134(2):229-236.

52. Reichenberger F, Voswinckel R, Enke B, et al. Long-term treatment with sildenafil in chronic thromboembolic pulmonary hypertension. *Eur Respir J*. 2007;30(5):922-927.

12 Pulmonary Hypertension in the ICU

by Steven Y. Chang, MD, PhD

Introduction

The development of specific therapies for the treatment of PAH has significantly improved the outcome of this disease.[1] Given the improvement in survival, it has become more likely that patients with PAH will, at some point, need admission to an intensive care unit (ICU). Robust, well-done studies of critically ill patients with PH are lacking. Even large interventional studies looking at the management of critical illnesses, such as sepsis and the acute respiratory distress syndrome (ARDS), rarely provide subgroup analysis of patients with pulmonary vascular disease. Because of the limited placebo-controlled evidence, the recommendations in this chapter are based primarily on the expert opinions of the author regarding the approach to critically ill patients with PH.

Acute Pulmonary Hypertension

The pulmonary circulation is a high-capacitance, low-resistance system. As a result, the right ventricle (RV) has evolved to be highly efficient in its role, as it has the same cardiac output as the left ventricle (LV) despite having one sixth of the muscle mass while performing one fourth of the work of the LV. The primary function of the RV is to maintain a low right atrial (RA) pressure to ensure adequate venous return and to provide constant low-pressure perfusion throughout the pulmonary vasculature. Like the LV, stroke volume (SV) of the RV is governed by preload, afterload, myocardial contractility, and heart rate. Unlike the LV, however, isovolumic contraction and relaxation are essentially nonexistent for the RV under normal conditions (**Figure 12.1**). Low right ventricular wall tensions allow coronary perfusion to occur during both systole and diastole unlike in the LV, where coronary perfusion only occurs during diastole because of the high wall tensions that are presents during systolic contraction.

It is generally accepted that in patients without pre-existing PH, the RV is capable of generating mean pressures of only about 40 mm Hg.[2] In conditions of acutely increased afterload, the RV dilates in order to

FIGURE 12.1 — Effect of Ventricular Volume Changes on Pressures in Right and Left Ventricles

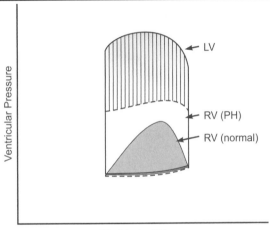

Under normal conditions, right ventricular isovolumic contraction and relaxation are nonexistent, right ventricle (RV) wall tensions are low, and coronary perfusion occurs throughout both systole and diastole *(shaded area)*. When the RV adapts in the face of elevated afterload such as is seen in pulmonary hypertension (PH), RV wall tensions increase such that coronary blood flow only occurs during diastole, and the RV pressure-volume loop starts to look like the left ventricle (LV) pressure-volume loop *(white area)*. A left ventricular press-volume loop is shown for comparison *(line-filled area)*.

maintain stroke volume and the ejection fraction (EF) is often decreased. RV wall tension can increase to the point where coronary blood flow only occurs during diastole (similar to the LV). Decreased coronary blood flow during systole can contribute to diminished RV performance (**Figure 12.1**).

The fates of the right and left ventricles are entwined because of the interventricular septum and the pericardium (**Figure 12.2**).[3] The load on each of the ventricles is dependent on the passive filling of the other. With increased RV afterload and RV end-diastolic volume, the interventricular septum shifts into the LV during diastole because of restrictions imposed by the pericardium, thus impairing left ventricular filling and function. Cardiac output and systemic perfusion then decrease, resulting in decreased RV perfusion and further worsening RV function (**Figure 12.3**).[4,5]

Common etiologies of acute right heart failure from acute PH include severe hypoxemic respiratory failure (ie, ARDS), massive PE, air/amniotic/fat/tumor emboli, pulmonary leukostasis/leukoagglutination, and sickle cell sludging. Positive pressure ventilation with high intrathoracic pressures can also result in acute RV failure (**Table 12.1**). Management strategies for ARDS and PE have resulted from large, randomized trials that were not likely to include a significant number of subjects with pre-existing PH.[6-11] Application of these principles to the critically ill PH patient is potentially problematic as patients with pre-existing PH have chronically adapted to persistent elevation of RV afterload, and the expected clinical responses to these therapies are not well known in these patients.

Triggers of RV failure from acute-on-chronic PH include those listed above for acute PH, and also include sepsis, anemia, trauma, surgery, dysrhythmias, pregnancy, and interruption of PH therapies (**Table 12.1**).[12] In addition to identifying triggers of worsening clinical status in order to rapidly address them, it is also absolutely critical to have a grasp of the PH patient's volume status.

12

FIGURE 12.2 — Inter-relationship of Right and Left Ventricular Volume

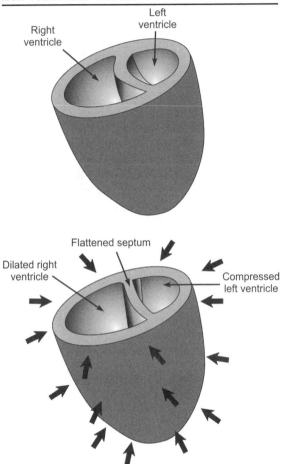

Because of the pericardium and interventricular septum, the right and left ventricles are interconnected. The load on one ventricle is dependent on the passive filling of the other. With high right ventricular afterloads and increased volume, the interventricular septum impinges on the left ventricle, and left ventricle filling and function are thus impacted.

Estimation of Volume Status and Fluid Responsiveness

Estimation of intravascular volume status is fraught with difficulty. For decades, the central venous pressure (CVP) has been used to guide volume resuscitation.[13] Recommendations for resuscitation in severe sepsis and septic shock include targeting a CVP of 8-12 mm Hg.[14,15] It has been assumed that because CVP reflects right atrial pressures and presumably right ventricular filling pressures, it would be a reasonable surrogate for RV preload and that increasing CVP would increase RV output and thus, cardiac output. However, CVP does not always correlate with overall volume state, RV end-diastolic volume, stroke volume, and thus, response to fluid challenges. The belief that CVP tracks RV filling pressures and preload responsiveness depends on problematic assumptions. Because of the nonlinear shape of the pressure-volume curve of the ventricles, the relationship between filling pressures and preload cannot be reliably predicted.[16,17]

The relationship between CVP and volume responsiveness in patients with PH may be even more difficult to gauge, especially with an already overloaded RV. Several well-done studies have either shown no benefit or worse outcome in critically ill patients managed with use of a pulmonary artery catheter (PAC).[18,19] However, these studies did not include patients with pre-existing PH. Intriguingly, a retrospective review of patients at a referral center for PH by Huynh and colleagues demonstrated that early placement of a PAC and incorporating its use in medical management improved survival in a group of patients with PH admitted to the ICU.[20]

Goal-directed echocardiography (GDE) is an alternative to static intravascular pressure measurements and may be useful for qualitative assessment of causes of hemodynamic instability and determination of whether a patient will respond to volume infusion.[21,22] If reasonably good windows can be obtained, right

12

243

FIGURE 12.3 — Pathophysiology of Right Ventricular Failure in the Context of Acute PH

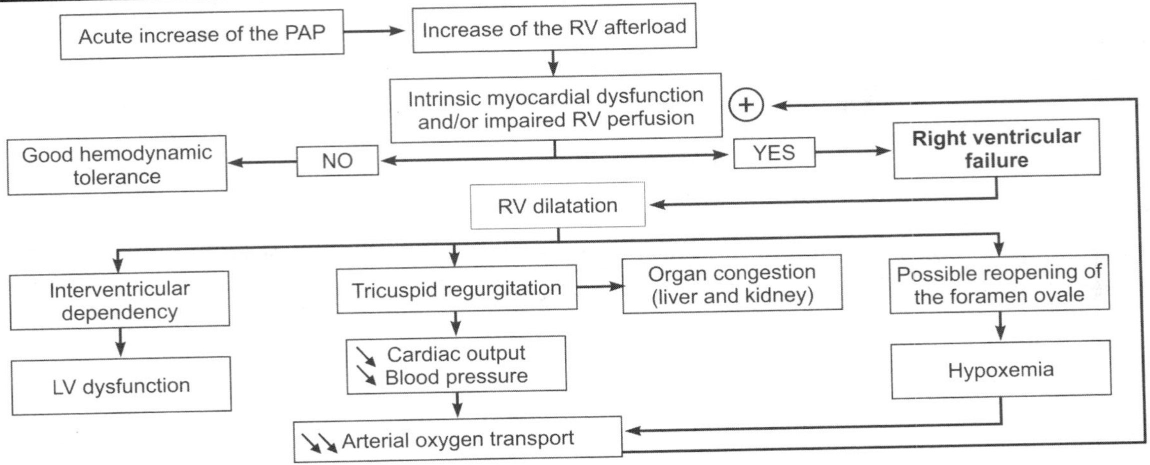

Progressive pulmonary hypertension and resultant increased right ventricular afterload results in RV dysfunction. Because of ventricular interdependence, left ventricular function is negatively impacted with resultant low cardiac output and cardiovascular collapse.

Gayat E, Mebazaa A. *Curr Opin Crit Care.* 2011;17(5):439-448.

12

TABLE 12.1 — Causes of Right Heart Failure

Acute Right Heart Failure
- Severe hypoxemic respiratory failure (eg, ARDS)
- Submassive-to-massive pulmonary embolism
- Air/amniotic/fat/tumor emboli
- Pulmonary leukostasis/leukoagglutination
- Sickle cell sludging
- Aggressive positive pressure ventilation (large tidal volumes, high PEEP)

Acute Right Heart Failure in Setting of Chronic PH
- Etiologies listed for acute right heart failure
- Sepsis
- Anemia
- Trauma
- Surgery
- Dysrhythmias
- Pregnancy
- Interruption of PH therapies

ventricular size and function can be assessed. While there are no reliable parameters for predicting patient response to volume, extremes of ventricular size can be useful. Underfilled and hyperdynamic ventricles are likely to predict good response to volume challenge, whereas overdistended ventricles with decreased systolic function are more likely to benefit from volume reduction. An estimate of volume responsiveness can also be gleaned from looking at the respiratory variation of the inferior vena cava (IVC). Variations in diameter of <12% suggest that patient hemodynamics will not improve with volume resuscitation, whereas variations of >18% suggest that patient hemodynamics will improve with fluid.[23-25] While static measurements of IVC diameter have not generally been shown to be as useful, they can still be of help in some patients. For instance, if the IVC diameter is <1 cm, it is likely that patients will be volume responsive, and if the IVC diameter is >2.5 cm, it is unlikely that patients will respond with hemodynamic improvement to IV fluid boluses, but response in patients with IVC diameters of 1 to 2.5 cm are unpredictable.[22]

For patients with PH, echocardiography is most useful in viewing the geometric relationship between the right and the left ventricle. Right ventricular dilation can be defined as a ratio of the RV end-diastolic area to LV end-diastolic area of >0.6 on a parasternal short-axis view or on an apical four-chamber view.[26] When faced with patients with overloaded RVs, it is unlikely that they will respond appropriately to volume resuscitation, and in fact, they would be more likely to benefit from diuresis and vasoactive support *(see below)*.

In nonpulmonary hypertensive patients with sepsis who are mechanically ventilated, pulse pressure variation (PPV) of >13% during the respiratory cycle can also predict a good response to volume infusion.[27] In order to perform the necessary measurements, however, patients need to be intubated and mechanically ventilated in passive fashion with tidal volumes (V_T) of 8-12 mL/kg of measured body weight, well above currently recommended lung protective settings. While this has been shown to be a reasonably good strategy for determining the response to the administration of IV fluids in septic patients who are mechanically ventilated, PPV is not reliable in patients with PH.[28] In fact, in many patients with PH, volume challenge was associated with reduced RV ejection fraction, likely due to overdistension of the RV as described above.

Resuscitation and Vasoactive Support

Both hypovolemia and hypervolemia can contribute to shock in patients with right ventricular dysfunction. Initial management of the PH patient with shock is determined by volume status. In cases in which patients are hypovolemic, judicious volume resuscitation is warranted, with frequent reassessment of volume state and responsiveness. Patients with RV dysfunction or failure can easily be tipped into a volume overloaded state with resultant decreased LV filling and cardiac output resulting in persistent shock.

When patients are hypervolemic with an overloaded RV and underfilled LV, aggressive diuresis is warranted in an attempt to normalize right ventricular and thus left ventricular function. If patients have renal dysfunction, renal replacement therapy to remove volume may be required.

If an adequate perfusion pressure cannot be achieved with manipulation of volume status, vasoactive support is required. It is important to keep systemic arterial pressure greater than RV systolic pressure so that RV perfusion from coronary blood flow is maintained throughout the cardiac cycle. Kwak and associates compared the hemodynamic effects of norepinephrine and phenylephrine in 27 subjects undergoing cardiac surgery with WHO Group 2 PH.[29] Norepinephrine was shown to be preferable to phenylephrine in patients with PH related to chronic left heart disease as it decreased the ratio of the mPAP to the mean systemic arterial pressures (MAP) while maintaining cardiac output. Norepinephrine is generally considered a good choice as an initial pressor to treat systemic hypotension in the critically ill patients with RV failure and/or PAH. Phenylephrine, on the other hand, did not decrease the MPAP:MAP ratio and had negative inotropic effects. Care must be taken, however, in extrapolating these results to the general PH patient population as this study was performed in Group 2 PH patients optimized for cardiac surgery. Vasopressin, a nonadrenergic vasoconstrictor, might be useful as it seems to reduce both PVR and the ratio of the PVR to the systemic vascular resistance (SVR).[30] Vasopressin has been safely used in severe sepsis/septic shock, although its mortality benefit is less certain.[31]

If optimization of volume status and correction of systemic hypotension fail to improve cardiac output, inotropic support may be needed. Dobutamine acts through β_1-adrenergic receptors to increase myocardial contractility and to decrease LV afterload.[5] In canine and leporine models, it decreased PVR at low doses (≤ 5 mcg/kg/min) while also augmenting output.[5,32,33]

At higher doses, dobutamine did not improve hemodynamics. Dopamine acts through adrenergic and dopaminergic receptors, but it should be used with care in patients with PH because of its hypotensive effects on the systemic circulation and propensity to increase tachyarrhythmias relative to other agents.[14,34] In PAH patients with RV failure, dobutamine is usually given at low doses from 2.5-5.0 ug/min and adjusted slowly while monitoring its effects on heart rate, blood pressure and cardiac output. Milrinone is a phosphodiesterase-3 inhibitor that acts as both an inotrope and a vasodilator which can reduce PAPs and RV afterload. Milrinone is a reasonable alternative to dobutamine for ionotropic support in critically ill patients with PAH, but patients must be monitored closely for systemic hypotension.

Nitric Oxide and Other Pulmonary Vasodilators

Pulmonary vasodilators currently approved for the treatment of PH are described in detail in *Chapters 6-9*. We will review salient features relevant to the management of the critically ill PH patient.

Inhaled nitric oxide (iNO) increases cGMP, dilating the pulmonary vasculature only in the regions into which it is inhaled, thereby preferentially vasodilating regions of the lung that are ventilated, thus improving oxygenation. Because it is rapidly inactivated by hemoglobin in the pulmonary capillaries, it does not lower systemic blood pressure. While iNO has been shown to have salutary effects on hemodynamic parameters in patients with right ventricular dysfunction and elevated PAPs, it is unclear whether it would positively impact survival in the critically ill patient with pre-existing PH. Certainly, it has *not* been shown to positively impact survival in ARDS, and it may even result in an increased incidence of acute kidney injury.[35,36]

The role of advanced therapies (prostanoids, endothelin receptor blockers, PDE5 inhibitors) in acutely

12

critically ill patients with PH is uncertain, although intravenous epoprostenol (prostacyclin [PGI_2]) has been shown to have mortality benefit in patients with NYHA class III or IV idiopathic pulmonary artery hypertension.[37] In a meta-analysis of 21 trials comparing various advanced PH therapies (eg, prostanoids, endothelin receptor blockers, PDE5 inhibitors, and the thromboxane synthase inhibitor, terbogrel) to placebo, Galie and colleagues found a RR of 0.57 (95% CI 0.35-0.93) for death. Initiation of these therapies could be difficult as the critically ill patient is often hypotensive and, with the exception of iNO, these therapies not only lower PAPs and PVR, but also lower MAP and SVR.[1] In general, PAH patients who have been taking pulmonary vasodilator medications should stay on them when they become critically ill. Stopping or reducing pulmonary vasodilatory therapy in a PAH patient who is hemodynamically unstable would not be expected improve their condition. Rather, patients should be kept on their medications in an attempt to reduce RV afterload while optimizing RV filling pressure and managing systemic hypotension with vasopressors.

For newly diagnosed PH or patients who require more aggressive pulmonary vasodilator therapy, new PAH-specific medications may be indicated. In this situation, the ideal agent would have a rapid onset of action, high degree of selectivity for the pulmonary circulation, and a short-half life. iNO or inhaled epoprostenol fit these characteristics best. Both agents are potent pulmonary vasodilators that act within minutes of being used. The inhalational route also avoids systemic hypotension or worsening of the alveolar-arterial O_2 gradient. Intravenous epoprostenol or sildenafil also have rapid onset of action and fairly short half-life but are more likely to cause systemic hypotension and worsen oxygenation. Oral pulmonary vasodilators, such as phosphodiesterase inhibitors, endothelin receptor antagonists, or the recently approved soluble guanylate cyclase stimulator riociguat, are best avoided in the critically ill patient because of their longer half-life and reduced selectivity for the pulmonary circulation.

When the decision is made to use or escalate advanced PH therapies, careful hemodynamic and oxygenation monitoring is required. It is important to correct any underlying conditions that can increase pulmonary vasoconstriction. Alveolar hypoxia and reduced oxygen tension in pulmonary arterial blood cause pulmonary vasoconstriction and can increase RV afterload significantly. For any level of hypoxia, pulmonary vasoconstriction is increased in the presence of academia or hypercapnia, and these abnormalities should be reversed if at all possible.

Acute Respiratory Failure

Right ventricular afterload is increased with institution of positive pressure ventilation via an increase in Zone 1 and Zone II lung (**Figure 12.4**), and has been shown to result in acute cor pulmonale and tricuspid regurgitation.[38,39] At the same time, the increase in intrathoracic pressure decreases right ventricular transmural filling pressure and thereby reduces right ventricular preload. Mechanical ventilatory strategies continue to evolve. Prior to the evolution of lung protective ventilation (LPV), more attention was paid to patient comfort, oxygenation, and pH. Commonly employed ventilator strategies using V_T of 10-15 mL/kg of measured body weight resulted in a rate of acute cor pulmonale of 61%.[38]

With institution of lower tidal volumes, the rate of acute cor pulmonale decreased to 25%.[39] However, in patients with PAH, the rate of RV failure is likely to be much higher. In general, patients with PAH tolerate positive pressure poorly when they are critically ill and most experts recommend avoiding intubation and mechanical ventilation if at all possible. If positive pressure ventilation is unavoidable, adapting a lung protective strategy in PH patients will likely benefit their hemodynamics, although care must be taken to avoid severe hypercapnia. Elevated pCO_2 has been shown to increase PAPs,[40,41] so if PH patients are

12

FIGURE 12.4 — The Effect of Ventricular Pressure on V/Q Relationships in the Lung

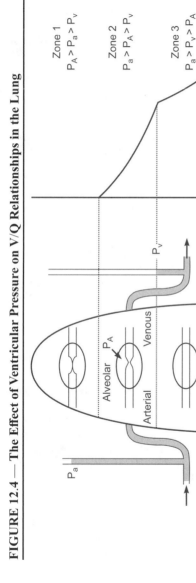

Zone 1
$P_A > P_a > P_v$

Zone 2
$P_a > P_A > P_v$

Zone 3
$P_a > P_v > P_A$

Blood flow

P_v

Alveolar P_A

Venous

Arterial

P_a

Aggressive positive pressure ventilation results in increased alveolar pressures which results in increased Zone I and Zone II lung. This results in increased right ventricular afterload.

instituted on appropriate ventilatory strategies, minute ventilation must be kept adequate in order to ensure relative normocapnia and acid-base status. Oxygen saturation should be kept at >92% to avoid hypoxic pulmonary vasoconstriction.

The benefits and effects of positive end-expiratory pressure (PEEP) are less clear. It is doubtful that in patients with chronic PH that empiric application of higher than physiologic PEEP (~5 cm H_2O) would be helpful, and it is likely to worsen hemodynamic variables by increasing right ventricular afterload and decreasing preload. The benefits and effects of PEEP on oxygenation must be weighed against its effects on hemodynamics. PEEP helps in recruiting alveoli and in some circumstances may be necessary to maintain oxygenation, which would result in less hypoxic vasoconstriction, thus resulting in decreased PVR.

A reasonable strategy for the intubated and mechanically ventilated PH patient would be to adopt a low V_T strategy and to use the minimum amount of PEEP necessary to maintain oxygenation adequate to keep the pulmonary vasculature vasodilated. The use of noninvasive positive pressure ventilation such as BIPAP and CPAP carries the same risk of adverse effect on right ventricular afterload and preload as endotracheal intubation but can often be used with less sedation. Still, these modalities are often not well tolerated in critically ill patients with PAH. The poor outcome of hemodynamically unstable PAH treated with positive pressure ventilation has led some intensivists to consider the use of extracorporeal life support in these patients when they develop respiratory failure (see section on *Rescue Therapies* below).

Dysrhythmias

Supraventricular tachyarrhythmias (SVT) seem to be especially detrimental in patients with PH. Because the dysfunctional RV is dependent on effective atrial contractility, maintenance of sinus rhythm can be critical.[12,42,43] In a single center, retrospective study, Tongers and associates found that mortality for PH patients was only 6.3% at approximately 2 years when sinus rhythm could be restored and maintained in PAH patients who developed SVT. However, 9 of 11 patients in whom sinus rhythm could not be maintained died during a follow-up period of 11 ± 8 months.[43] A single center review of 82 consecutive patients with sepsis and non-Group 2 PH revealed that new onset atrial fibrillation was a strong predictor of increased hospital mortality (OR 6.51; 95% CI 2.24-22.07).[44] The acute onset of SVT should be treated aggressively in critically ill patients with PAH. The use of electrocardioversion is often necessary to restore sinus rhythm and some patients will require pharmacologic therapy after cardioversion to prevent recurrence of SVT.

Trauma

A 2013 retrospective review of 187 trauma patients showed that PH did not predict mortality in the trauma population.[45] PH was arbitrarily defined as a PASP of >45 mm Hg, and a subset of patients with PASP >60 mm Hg was prespecified. A total of 39 of 187 patients were found to have PH by this definition. Mortality for controls and PH patients was 25.6% and 26.4%, respectively ($P = 1.0$). The nine patients with PASP >60 mm Hg, however, had a mortality 44% compared with 25.3% for the controls ($P = 0.2444$).

Sepsis

ICU mortality in PH patients ranges from 30% to 41% compared with a mortality of 10.8% in the general ICU population.[20,46,47] In two retrospective reviews of critically ill PH patients, sepsis was found to significantly worsen outcomes.[20,47] In fact, sepsis increased the odds of dying more than any other factor (OR 14.0 [2.42-80.9]; $P < 0.03$).[20] Sepsis worsens both right and left ventricular function,[48] and in patients with an already compromised RV, this can be deleterious. In any patient with sepsis, it is important to identify offending organisms when possible. Appropriate broad-spectrum antibiotics should be rapidly administered and drainage of infected sources should be performed whenever possible. Careful attention to fluid resuscitation is necessary, given that many PH patients are already volume overloaded, and volume status and responsiveness must be frequently assessed. If PH patients appear to be volume overloaded, they may benefit from diuresis so that RV preload is decreased, allowing improved LV filling and improved cardiac output. In cases in which PH patients remain in shock, vasoactive support can be instituted with the caveats noted (see *Resuscitation and Vasoactive Support*).

Predictors of poor outcome in non-Group 2 PH patients with severe sepsis or septic shock include the severity of PH, acute-onset atrial fibrillation, and prolonged duration of vasoactive support.[44]

Rescue Therapies

If the more conventional approaches to resuscitating and stabilizing critically ill patients with PH do not work, atrial septostomy might be a palliative option or bridge to lung transplantation.[49] It has been noted that patients with Eisenmenger syndrome have better survival than patients with pulmonary artery hypertension.[49,50] As such, atrial septostomy can help to unload the RV, allowing for increased cardiac output. It is currently, however, not a proven strategy and is considered to be palliative.[49] Alternatively, critically ill PH patients awaiting lung or heart-lung transplant who do not respond to aggressive medical therapy might be started on invasive mechanical support such as veno-arterial extracorporeal membrane oxygenation (V-A ECMO),[51] right ventricular assist devices (RVADs),[52] or even devices which entirely bypass the right heart by connecting the pulmonary artery to the left atrium with a membrane oxygenator.[53] Although these therapies are

12

generally reserved as a bridge to lung transplantation, there have been reports of ECMO being used as a bridge to recovery in critically ill patients with PAH.[54] Finally, lung or heart-lung transplantation can be pursued if all other options are exhausted and the patient is otherwise an appropriate candidate.[49]

Outcomes

Despite recent advances in medical therapy, PAH remains a progressive disease without a cure. Unfortunately, the majority of PAH patients who succumb to their disease do not die at home in comfortable and familiar settings but appear to require critical care medicine. In a survey of surrogates of 36 PAH patients who recently died, Grinnan and colleagues found that 90% of deaths were due to PAH itself, that most patients died in the hospital (67%), and that most of the deaths in the hospital occurred in the ICU (83%).[55] Tonelli and coworkers reviewed, in prospective fashion, 84 PAH patient deaths, finding that PH was either the direct cause or played a role in death in 74 of these patients. A total of 74 of 84 patients died in a health care setting with 42 of those patients dying in an ICU.[56] Clearly, being in a hospital does not prevent death, and in fact, Hoeper and associates report that nearly 80% of PAH patients who undergo CPR *in a hospital setting* do not survive.[57] As more patients are diagnosed with and treated for PAH, the number of patients with PAH who present to the ICU is likely to increase. Considering their unique requirements for maintaining right ventricular output in the setting of increased cardiac demand and decreased systemic vascular resistance, these patients are likely to represent a unique population that requires further study.

- In patients with PH who are hemodynamically unstable, accurate assessment of intravascular volume status is essential to their management as they may require either volume administration or diuresis. Administration of volume to an already overloaded patient can worsen their hemodynamics.
- Static measures of intravascular pressures such as CVP may not be reliable indicators of volume status. A more reasonable alternative may be the use GDE.
- Factors that contribute to increased PVR such as hypoxia, hypercapnia, and academia should be reversed or controlled to the extent possible.
- Systemic arterial pressure must be kept greater than pulmonary systolic pressure to maintain right ventricular perfusion. Norepinephrine or dobutamine are reasonable choices for initial vasopressor and inotropic support.
- Positive pressure ventilation can worsen RV function by increasing afterload and decreasing preload, and should be avoided if at all possible.
- Selective pulmonary vasodilators should be considered in an attempt to acutely lower PVR. Inhaled pulmonary vasodilators such as nitric oxide or nebulized epoprostenol have the greatest selectivity for the pulmonary vascular bed and the least effect on worsening oxygenation.
- PAH patients admitted to the ICU have a poor prognosis with sepsis being the most common cause of ICU mortality.

12

REFERENCES

1. Galiè N, Manes A, Negro L, Palazzini M, Bacchi-Reggiani ML, Branzi A. A meta-analysis of randomized controlled trials in pulmonary arterial hypertension. *Eur Heart J*. 2009;30(4):394-403.

2. Chin KM, Kim NH, Rubin LJ. The right ventricle in pulmonary hypertension. *Coron Artery Dis*. 2005;16(1):13-18.

3. Dell'Italia LJ. Reperfusion for right ventricular infarction. *N Engl J Med*. 1998;338(14):978-980.

4. Gayat E, Mebazaa A. Pulmonary hypertension in critical care. *Curr Opin Crit Care*. 2011;17(5):439-448.

5. Zamanian RT, Haddad F, Doyle RL, Weinacker AB. Management strategies for patients with pulmonary hypertension in the intensive care unit. *Crit Care Med*. 2007;35(9):2037-2050.

6. Ventilation with lower tidal volumes as compared with traditional tidal volumes for acute lung injury and the acute respiratory distress syndrome. The Acute Respiratory Distress Syndrome Network. *N Engl J Med*. 2000;342(18):1301-1308.

7. Hamel E, Pacouret G, Vincentelli D, et al. Thrombolysis or heparin therapy in massive pulmonary embolism with right ventricular dilation: results from a 128-patient monocenter registry. *Chest*. 2001;120(1):120-125.

8. Konstantinides S, Geibel A, Heusel G, Heinrich F, Kasper W; Management Strategies and Prognosis of Pulmonary Embolism-3 Trial Investigators. Heparin plus alteplase compared with heparin alone in patients with submassive pulmonary embolism. *N Engl J Med*. 2002;347(15):1143-1150.

9. Meade MO, Cook DJ, Guyatt GH, et al; Lung Open Ventilation Study Investigators. Ventilation strategy using low tidal volumes, recruitment maneuvers, and high positive end-expiratory pressure for acute lung injury and acute respiratory distress syndrome: a randomized controlled trial. *JAMA*. 2008;299(6):637-645.

10. Meyer G, Vicaut E, Danays T, et al; PEITHO Investigators. Fibrinolysis for patients with intermediate-risk pulmonary embolism. *N Engl J Med*. 2014;370(15):1402-1411.

11. Stein PD, Matta F. Thrombolytic therapy in unstable patients with acute pulmonary embolism: saves lives but underused. *Am J Med*. 2012;125(5):465-470.

12. Hoeper MM, Granton J. Intensive care unit management of patients with severe pulmonary hypertension and right heart failure. *Am J Respir Crit Care Med*. 2011;184(10):1114-1124.

13. Wilson JN, Grow JB, Demong CV, Prevedel AE, Owens JC. Central venous pressure in optimal blood volume maintenance. *Arch Surg*. 1962;85:563-578.

14. Dellinger RP, Levy MM, Rhodes A, et al; Surviving Sepsis Campaign Guidelines Committee including the Pediatric Subgroup. Surviving sepsis campaign: international guidelines for management of severe sepsis and septic shock: 2012. *Crit Care Med*. 2013;41(2):580-637.

15. Rivers E, Nguyen B, Havstad S, et al; Early Goal-Directed Therapy Collaborative Group. Early goal-directed therapy in the treatment of severe sepsis and septic shock. *N Engl J Med*. 2001;345(19):1368-1377.

16. Marik PE, Cavallazzi R. Does the central venous pressure predict fluid responsiveness? An updated meta-analysis and a plea for some common sense. *Crit Care Med*. 2013;41(7):1774-1781.

17. Osman D, Ridel C, Ray P, et al. Cardiac filling pressures are not appropriate to predict hemodynamic response to volume challenge. *Crit Care Med*. 2007;35(1):64-68.

18. Connors AF Jr, Speroff T, Dawson NV, et al. The effectiveness of right heart catheterization in the initial care of critically ill patients. SUPPORT Investigators. *JAMA*. 1996;276(11):889-897.

19. Wheeler AP, Bernard GR, Thompson BT et al; National Heart, Lung, and Blood Institute Acute Respiratory Distress Syndrome (ARDS) Clinical Trials Network. Pulmonary-artery versus central venous catheter to guide treatment of acute lung injury. *N Engl J Med*. 2006;354(21):2213-2224.

20. Huynh TN, Weigt SS, Sugar CA, Shapiro S, Kleerup EC. Prognostic factors and outcomes of patients with pulmonary hypertension admitted to the intensive care unit. *J Crit Care*. 2012;27(6):739.e7-e13.

21. Repessé X, Charron C, Vieillard-Baron A. Intensive care ultrasound: V. Goal-directed echocardiography. *Ann Am Thorac Soc*. 2014;11(1):122-128.

22. Schmidt GA, Koenig S, Mayo PH. Shock: ultrasound to guide diagnosis and therapy. *Chest*. 2012;142(4):1042-1048.

23. De Backer D, Fagnoul D. Intensive care ultrasound: VI. Fluid responsiveness and shock assessment. *Ann Am Thorac Soc*. 2014;11(1):129-136.

24. Barbier C, Loubières Y, Schmit C, et al. Respiratory changes in inferior vena cava diameter are helpful in predicting fluid responsiveness in ventilated septic patients. *Intensive Care Med*. 2004;30(9):1740-1746.

259

25. Feissel M, Michard F, Faller JP, Teboul JL. The respiratory variation in inferior vena cava diameter as a guide to fluid therapy. *Intensive Care Med.* 2004;30(9):1834-1837.

26. Jardin F, Dubourg O, Bourdarias JP. Echocardiographic pattern of acute cor pulmonale. *Chest.* 1997;111(1):209-217.

27. Michard F, Boussat S, Chemla D, et al. Relation between respiratory changes in arterial pulse pressure and fluid responsiveness in septic patients with acute circulatory failure. *Am J Respir Crit Care Med.* 2000;162(1):134-138.

28. Wyler von Ballmoos M, Takala J, Roeck M, et al. Pulse-pressure variation and hemodynamic response in patients with elevated pulmonary artery pressure: a clinical study. *Crit Care.* 2010;14(3):R111.

29. Kwak YL, Lee CS, Park YH, Hong YW. The effect of phenyl-ephrine and norepinephrine in patients with chronic pulmonary hypertension*. *Anaesthesia.* 2002;57(1):9-14.

30. Price LC, Wort SJ, Finney SJ, Marino PS, Brett SJ. Pulmonary vascular and right ventricular dysfunction in adult critical care: current and emerging options for management: a systematic literature review. *Crit Care.* 2010;14(5):R169.

31. Russell JA, Walley KR, Singer J, et al; VASST Investigators. Vasopressin versus norepinephrine infusion in patients with septic shock. *N Engl J Med.* 2008;358(9):877-887.

32. Bradford KK, Deb B, Pearl RG. Combination therapy with inhaled nitric oxide and intravenous dobutamine during pulmonary hypertension in the rabbit. *J Cardiovasc Pharmacol.* 2000;36(2):146-151.

33. Kerbaul F, Rondelet B, Motte S, et al. Effects of norepinephrine and dobutamine on pressure load-induced right ventricular failure. *Crit Care Med.* 2004;32(4):1035-1040.

34. De Backer D, Biston P, Devriendt J, et al; SOAP II Investigators. Comparison of dopamine and norepinephrine in the treatment of shock. *N Engl J Med.* 2010;362(9):779-789.

35. Taylor RW, Zimmerman JL, Dellinger RP, et al; Inhaled Nitric Oxide in ARDS Study Group. Low-dose inhaled nitric oxide in patients with acute lung injury: a randomized controlled trial. *JAMA.* 2004;291(13):1603-1609.

36. Adhikari NK, Burns KE, Friedrich JO, Granton JT, Cook DJ, Meade MO. Effect of nitric oxide on oxygenation and mortality in acute lung injury: systematic review and meta-analysis. *BMJ.* 2007;334(7597):779.

37. Barst RJ, Rubin LJ, Long WA, et al; Primary Pulmonary Hypertension Study Group. A comparison of continuous intravenous epoprostenol (prostacyclin) with conventional therapy for primary pulmonary hypertension. *N Engl J Med.* 1996;334(5):296-301.

38. Jardin F, Gueret P, Dubourg O, Farcot JC, Margairaz A, Bourdarias JP. Two-dimensional echocardiographic evaluation of right ventricular size and contractility in acute respiratory failure. *Crit Care Med.* 1985;13(11):952-956.

39. Vieillard-Baron A, Schmitt JM, Augarde R, et al. Acute cor pulmonale in acute respiratory distress syndrome submitted to protective ventilation: incidence, clinical implications, and prognosis. *Crit Care Med.* 2001;29(8):1551-1555.

40. Carvalho CR, Barbas CS, Medeiros DM, et al. Temporal hemodynamic effects of permissive hypercapnia associated with ideal PEEP in ARDS. *Am J Respir Crit Care Med.* 1997;156(5):1458-1466.

41. Thorens JB, Jolliet P, Ritz M, Chevrolet JC. Effects of rapid permissive hypercapnia on hemodynamics, gas exchange, and oxygen transport and consumption during mechanical ventilation for the acute respiratory distress syndrome. *Intensive Care Med.* 1996;22(3):182-191.

42. Goldstein JA, Harada A, Yagi Y, Barzilai B, Cox JL. Hemo-dynamic importance of systolic ventricular interaction, aug-mented right atrial contractility and atrioventricular synchrony in acute right ventricular dysfunction. *J Am Coll Cardiol.* 1990;16(1):181-189.

43. Tongers J, Schwerdtfeger B, Klein G, et al. Incidence and clinical relevance of supraventricular tachyarrhythmias in pulmonary hypertension. *Am Heart J.* 2007;153(1):127-132.

44. Tsapenko MV, Herasevich V, Mour GK, et al. Severe sepsis and septic shock in patients with pre-existing non-cardiac pulmo-nary hypertension: contemporary management and outcomes. *Crit Care Resusc.* 2013;15(2):103-109.

45. Friend KE, Britt R, Collins J, Novosel T, Weireter L. Pul-monary hypertension is not an independent risk factor for morbidity and mortality in the trauma population. *Am Surg.* 2013;79(7):743-745.

46. Checkley W, Martin GS, Brown SM, et al; United States Criti-cal Illness and Injury Trials Group Critical Illness Outcomes Study Investigators. Structure, process, and annual ICU mortal-ity across 69 centers: United States Critical Illness and Injury Trials Group Critical Illness Outcomes Study. *Crit Care Med.* 2014;42(2):344-356.

12

47. Sztrymf B, Souza R, Bertoletti L, et al. Prognostic factors of acute heart failure in patients with pulmonary arterial hypertension. *Eur Respir J*. 2010;35(6):1286-1293.

48. Parker MM, McCarthy KE, Ognibene FP, Parrillo JE. Right ventricular dysfunction and dilatation, similar to left ventricular changes, characterize the cardiac depression of septic shock in humans. *Chest*. 1990;97(1):126-131.

49. Keogh AM, Mayer E, Benza RL, et al. Interventional and surgical modalities of treatment in pulmonary hypertension. *J Am Coll Cardiol*. 2009;54(1 Suppl):S67-S77.

50. Hopkins WE, Ochoa LL, Richardson GW, Trulock EP. Comparison of the hemodynamics and survival of adults with severe primary pulmonary hypertension or Eisenmenger syndrome. *J Heart Lung Transplant*. 1996;15(1 Pt 1):100-105.

51. Gregoric ID, Chandra D, Myers TJ, Scheinin SA, Loyalka P, Kar B. Extracorporeal membrane oxygenation as a bridge to emergency heart-lung transplantation in a patient with idiopathic pulmonary arterial hypertension. *J Heart Lung Transplant*. 2008;27(4):466-468.

52. Punnoose L, Burkhoff D, Rich S, Horn EM. Right ventricular assist device in end-stage pulmonary arterial hypertension: insights from a computational model of the cardiovascular system. *Prog Cardiovasc Dis*. 2012;55(2):234-243.e2.

53. Strueber M, Hoeper MM, Fischer S, et al. Bridge to thoracic organ transplantation in patients with pulmonary arterial hypertension using a pumpless lung assist device. *Am J Transplant*. 2009;9(4):853-857.

54. Rosenzweig EB, Brodie D, Abrams DC, Agerstrand CL, Bacchetta M. Extracorporeal membrane oxygenation as a novel bridging strategy for acute right heart failure in group 1 pulmonary arterial hypertension. *ASAIO J*. 2014;60(1):129-133.

55. Grinnan DC, Swetz KM, Pinson J, Fairman P, Lyckholm LJ, Smith T. The end-of-life experience for a cohort of patients with pulmonary arterial hypertension. *J Palliat Med*. 2012;15(10):1065-1070.

56. Tonelli AR, Arelli V, Minai OA, et al. Causes and circumstances of death in pulmonary arterial hypertension. *Am J Respir Crit Care Med*. 2013;188(3):365-369.

57. Hoeper MM, Galié N, Murali S, et al. Outcome after cardiopulmonary resuscitation in patients with pulmonary arterial hypertension. *Am J Respir Crit Care Med*. 2002;165(3):341-344.

13 Pulmonary Hypertension in the Pediatric Patient

by Hussam Inany, MD and
Pramod Narula, MD

Introduction

The hemodynamic criteria for PH in infants and children is the same as it is in adults. PH is defined as a mean pulmonary arterial pressure (mPAP) ≥25 mm Hg.[1] The underlying cause of PH in children differs from that of adult PH patients in that most cases are due to IPAH, HPAH, or congenital heart disease. Early detection and treatment may prevent disease progression. The prognosis depends on the underlying etiology and course of disease.

PH should be suspected in any child presenting with signs or symptoms suggesting heart failure (eg, shortness of breath, dyspnea on exertion, poor feeding, poor growth, or failure to thrive). Classification of the pulmonary hypertensive diseases is shown in **Table 1.1**. In the most recent revision of this classification scheme, persistent PH of the newborn has been made into a subcategory of WHO Group 1 PAH and congenital/acquired left heart inflow/outflow tract obstruction and congenital cardiomyopathies has been added to WHO Group 2.

Persistent Pulmonary Hypertension of the Newborn (PPHN)

■ Epidemiology and Etiology

PPHN occurs in 1.9 per 1000 live births and is associated with substantial morbidity and mortality.[2] The most common risk factor is meconium-stained amniotic fluid. PPHN can also be idiopathic or secondary to conditions such as birth asphyxia, respiratory distress syndrome, hypoglycemia, polycythemia, and pulmonary hypoplasia (eg, due to congenital diaphragmatic hernia).[3]

■ Pathophysiology

In utero, the pulmonary vascular resistance (PVR) is elevated relative to systemic pressure allowing shunting of oxygenated blood to the systemic circulation via the foramen ovale and ductus arteriosus.[4] After birth, numerous factors lead to a rapid decrease in PVR including the vasodilatory effects of lung inflation, an increase in alveolar O_2, increased PaO_2 and pH in pulmonary arterial blood and the release of prostaglandins and NO which act as local pulmonary vasodilators regulatory, and removal of the placenta.[3] If these changes do not achieve a significant drop in PVR, fetal circulation (right-to-left shunting via ductus arteriosus and foramen ovale) will persist after birth resulting in elevated PVR and the development of PH.

Maladaptation to normal fetal circulation transition after birth may occur due to meconium aspiration, imbalance in local vasodilatory and vasoconstrictor metabolites, chronic fetal hypoxia in utero leading to increased pulmonary artery medial muscle thickness, pulmonary hypoplasia (eg, as a complication of diaphragmatic hernia and/or oligohydramnios), and pulmonary vessels obstruction due to polycythemia.[3] All of these factors can increase the neonatal PVR and eventually the chance of development of PPHN.

■ Clinical Manifestations

Signs and symptoms vary according to the underlying etiology. Newborns with PPHN can present with cyanosis, signs of respiratory distress (eg, grunting, flaring, retractions, tachypnea), tachycardia, and shock.[3]

Auscultation of the heart may reveal a loud second heart sound and/or systolic murmur from tricuspid insufficiency.[1]

Diagnosis

Hypoxemia that does not improve substantially to 100% oxygen strongly suggests the presence of right to left shunt. In the absence of parenchymal or vascular lung disease this usually suggests an intracardiac shunt.

If right-to-left shunting through the ductus arteriosus is present the alveolar-arterial O_2 difference $(PAO_2 - PaO_2)$ will be >20 mm Hg.[3,4] A difference of >5% in O_2 saturation between preductal and postductal sites is an indication of shunting as well.[4]

Echocardiography with Doppler flow imaging studies may show right-to-left or bidirectional shunting across a patent foramen ovale and ductus arteriosus. Deviation of the atrial septum into the left atrium is seen in severe PPHN and tricuspid regurgitation can also be seen.[3]

The chest x-ray will usually be normal, but diminished vascular markings or cardiomegaly can be seen.[3] Dilated loops of bowel in left hemithorax indicate diaphragmatic hernia.

Treatment

Treatment goal is to prevent end-organ damage by correcting the underlying etiology, lowering PVR, and maintaining normal systemic pressure.[3]

Systemic arterial pressure can be maintained by fluid resuscitation and administering vasopressors.[3,4] Dopamine is the most frequently used agent. This will lead to a decrease in the pulmonary/systemic pressure gradient and reduces shunting and hypoxemia.[3]

Administering high concentrations of oxygen helps to lower PVR. If hypoxemia is not responding to high concentrations of oxygen (refractory hypoxemia), inhaled nitric oxide (iNO) can be used.[3] iNO diffuses across the alveolar epithelial and pulmonary vascular endothelial membranes into pulmonary vascular smooth muscle where it activates soluble guanylate cyclase and increases cGMP, resulting in vascular smooth muscle relaxation and vasodilatation.[3,4] In clinical trials, the use of iNO reduced the need for

13

extracorporeal membrane oxygenation (ECMO) support by approximately 40%.[3] Inhaled or intravenous prostacyclin (prostaglandin I_2) inhibits platelet aggregation and is also an effective vasodilator used for cases that do not respond to iNO.

Mechanical ventilation improves oxygenation by improving ventilation/perfusion and alveolar recruitment.[4] The use of mechanical ventilation can improve the efficacy of iNO if the newborn is suffering from parenchymal lung disease and decreases the need for ECMO. The use of surfactant in cases of surfactant deficiency (eg, meconium aspiration) reduces the need of ECMO as well.[4]

If the above treatments do not restore adequate oxygenation and circulation, ECMO provides cardiopulmonary support allowing time for heart, lungs, and vessels to recover.[3] An oxygenation index (mean airway pressure X $FiO_2 \times 100/PaO_2$) (OI) >40 predict a high mortality rate and is used to evaluate the need for using ECMO.[5]

Pulmonary Hypertension in Infants and Children

■ **Epidemiology and Etiology**

The incidence of PH in children varies depending on the child's age and the underlying etiology. Registries from the United Kingdom and the Netherlands report annual incidence rates of IPAH and PAH associated with congenital heart disease between 0.5 and 2.2 cases per million children.[6,7] IPAH, inherited PAH, and PAH associated with congenital heart disease are responsible for most of cases of pediatric PH,[8] and in one study[9] accounted for 93% of cases.

Congenital Heart Defect

Congenital heart defects can lead to PH via several mechanisms. When a congenital heart lesion creates a significant left-to-right shunt between the systemic and pulmonary circulation, increased shear pulmonary blood flow can result in remodeling of the pulmonary circulation and the development of PH. Left-to-right shunts can occur via intracardiac lesions, such as atrial or ventricular septal defects (ASD and VSD), or as extracardiac shunts, such as the persistence of patent ductus arteriosus.[3,10] This left-to-right shunt increases flow in the pulmonary vascular bed leading to changes in shear stress on the endothelial wall that lead to pulmonary arteriolar endothelial dysfunction and eventually hypertrophy of the arteriolar smooth muscle and/or proliferation of pulmonary vascular endothelial cells.[3]

Left heart disease or dysfunction such as mitral stenosis or left ventricular failure can also lead to the development of PH by increase pulmonary venous pressure.[3,11]

Eisenmenger Syndrome

As PH from a left-to-right shunt progresses, there may come a point when pulmonary pressure exceeds the systemic arterial pressure. At this point, the left-to-right shunt reverses, leading to right-to-left shunt.[3] Symptoms of right-to-left shunting such as hypoxemia, cyanosis, dyspnea, and fatigue usually develop gradually and do not manifest clinically until the second or third decade of life. As right-to-left shunting increases, patients will progress to right heart failure and develop headache, syncope, and hemoptysis. Early surgical intervention to repair the underlying congenital heart defect can prevent the development of PH and Eisenmenger syndrome.[3]

13

Idiopathic (Primary) Pulmonary Hypertension

IPAH, formerly known as primary PH, occurs when there is a progressive elevation in mPAP without a known etiology.[3,10] IPAH can occur at any age, but in children, the diagnosis is often made in adolescence. There is a female preponderance, with a female-to-male ratio of 1.7:1. Approximately 6% to 10% of cases are familial, and most of familial cases are caused by mutations in the gene for bone morphogenic protein receptor-2. The BMPR-2 gene mutations associated with HPAH are autosomal dominant primary pulmonary hypertension (PPH1).[3,10,12]

Although the cause of pulmonary vascular remodeling seen in IPAH and HPAH is not well understood, an imbalance in mediators of pulmonary vasodilatation and vasoconstriction has been observed. Most patients exhibit increase synthesis of the potent endothelial-derived vasoconstrictor endothelin-1 and decreased synthesis of the endogenous vasodilators prostacyclin and nitric oxide. Vascular remodeling with near or complete obliteration of a large number of distal pulmonary vessels occurs due to a proliferation of endothelial cells, vascular smooth muscle hypertrophy, and in situ thrombosis.[3,13,14]

Before a diagnosis of primary PH can be made, other causes of elevated PAP such as hypoxic lung disease, sleep disordered breathing, venous thromboembolism, or left-sided heart disease must be excluded.

Respiratory Disorders

Chronic hypoxic states (eg, living at high altitude) lead to hypoxic pulmonary vasoconstriction, medial hypertrophy, and increased muscularization of the small arteries. These changes are initially reversible if normoxia is restored, but chronic hypoxic exposure can lead to more permanent vascular remodeling and increased PVR.[3,13] Thoracic cage abnormalities (eg, kyphoscoliosis) and neuromuscular diseases (eg, muscular dystrophy, poliomyelitis, and myasthenia gravis) can lead to restrictive lung and alveolar hypoventilation and subsequent hypoxemia that can cause vasoconstriction and eventually PH.[3,15] Similarly, congenital central hypoventilation syndrome (CCHS) can lead to hypoxia-induced pulmonary vasoconstriction and PH.

Patients who have obstructive sleep apnea tend to have frequent episodes of oxygen desaturation that can lead to hypoxia-induced pulmonary vasoconstriction that results in elevation of PAP.[3,16]

Chronic gastroesophageal reflux disease (GERD) may cause interstitial fibrosis from chronic airway exposure to gastric acid[17] that can lead to PH.

Thromboembolic Disease

Chronic or recurrent venous thromboembolism causes pulmonary vascular obstruction and eventually can lead to the development of CTEPH (see *Chapter 11*).[3,8]

■ Presentation

Clinical Manifestation

Clinical manifestations in pediatric PH are related to the degree of PAP elevation and right ventricle dysfunction. Although there are different causes for PH, the clinical manifestations are nearly the same. Most patients will present with dyspnea on exertion that occurs because the right side of the heart is unable to adequately increase cardiac output with activities. Impairment of the right side of the heart may also manifest as tiring while feeding or failure to thrive. Syncope can occur in late stages of disease. Patients with severe right-to-left shunt may present with cyanosis. Other symptoms include chest pain, peripheral edema, and cardiac arrhythmias.[1,3,16] The symptoms of PH in infants and children is shown in **Table 13.1**.

TABLE 13.1 — Symptoms of Pulmonary Hypertension in Pediatric Patients

Infants	Children
• Cyanosis	• Dyspnea
• Failure to thrive	• Exercise intolerance
• Lethargy	• Chest pain
• Feeding difficulties	• Cyanosis
• Fussiness or irritability	• Edema
	• Abdominal distension

13

Diagnostic Studies

The diagnostic approach for PAH is shown in **Figure 13.1**.

- *EKG*: Classically will show signs of right ventricular hypertrophy, right axis deviation, and spiked P wave in lead II.[3,18,19]
- *Chest x-ray*: Will show signs of the underlying disease, enlargement of right ventricle, prominent hilar pulmonary arteries, and oligemic lung fields (decrease peripheral lung markings).[16,20]
- *Echocardiography:* Detects congenital heart defects. Right ventricular and right atrial enlargement may be seen. Doppler ultrasound can be used to evaluation right ventricular systolic pressure and left heart valvular function.[3,16,18]
- *Arterial blood gas*: Can detect hypoxia and acidosis.[18]
- *Ventilation perfusion scan:* Is helpful as a screening test for patients in whom CTEPH is suspected.[16,18]
- *Pulmonary angiography:* Performed if scan shows ventilation perfusion mismatch to exclude chronic thromboembolism.[16,18]
- *Pulmonary function test*: May help detect the underlying lung disease causing secondary PH (eg, restrictive and obstructive pulmonary diseases).[18]
- *Cardiac catheterization:* Is the gold standard for confirming the diagnosis of PAH and for guiding management. It can exclude the presence of pulmonary venous hypertension by measuring left-sided filling pressure.[1,18] Cardiac catheterization can also detect shunts, congenital heart diseases, and peripheral pulmonary artery stenosis.[1,18] Catheterization of the right heart is also necessary for acute vasodilator testing (AVT).[8]

■ Treatment

The ultimate goal of treatment is to improve survival and to allow normal activities of childhood. However, the endpoints used to assess response to treatment in children may differ from those used in adults. For example, normal values for 6MWD are less well established and the WHO functional class scheme used in adult patients was not designed to be used in children. Hemodynamic parameters correlate with prognosis, but the values differ from those used in adult patients.

Currently, the prognosis of children with PH has improved due to new therapeutic agents and the aggressive treatment strategies. Prior to the onset of modern medical therapies, survival of PAH in children was dismal and similar to that in adults. With the development of PAH-specific medications, long-term survival has improved. In the REVEAL registry from the United States, patients with childhood-onset PAH had a 1-, 3-, and 5-year estimated survival rate of $96 \pm 4\%$, $84 \pm 5\%$, and $74 \pm 6\%$, respectively, and no difference was seen between patients with IPAH ($75 \pm 7\%$) or PAH associated with congenital heart disease.[21] Identifying the etiology is the initial step in managing PH. Following the complete evaluation for all causes of PH, AVT is recommended to help determine therapy. The definition of an acute vasodilator response differs somewhat in pediatric patients. The criteria of a decrease in mPAP or >10 mm Hg to a mPAP <40 mm Hg is not as uniformly accepted as it is in adult patients as long-term response to CCBs has not been studied using this definition in children. Instead, the modified Barst criteria, defined as a 20% decrease in mPAP with normal or sustained cardiac output and no change or a decrease in the ratio of pulmonary to systemic vascular resistance (PVR/SVR) has been used to predict a sustained response to CCBs.[22]

Calcium Channel Blockers

Patients who demonstrate an acute pulmonary vasodilator response are most likely to benefit from

13

FIGURE 13.1 — Diagnostic Approach for Pediatric PAH

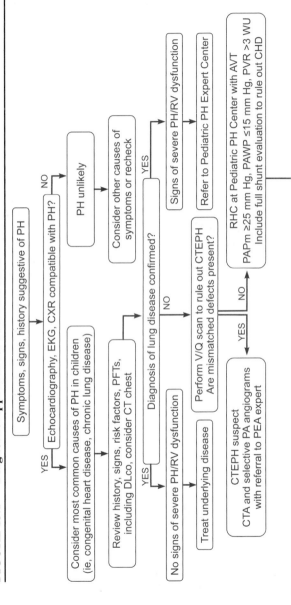

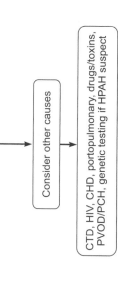

Consider other causes

CTD, HIV, CHD, portopulmonary, drugs/toxins, PVOD/PCH, genetic testing if HPAH suspect

13

273

treatment with CCBs such as amlodipine, nifedipine, or diltiazem.[1,8] In general, CCBs are not used in infants <1 year of age due to their negative inotropic effects.

For children with PAH who do not exhibit a positive pulmonary vasodilator response, the optimal therapeutic approach is not clear. The use of PAH-specific medications in children with PAH is based almost exclusively on clinical data that were derived from studies in adult patients. Due to substantial differences in the etiologies and the uncertainty of the most useful clinical endpoints in children, it has been difficult to determine selection of the most appropriate therapy. Recent guidelines have been developed by the WHO working group on pediatric PH at the 2013 World Symposium on Pulmonary Hypertension in Nice, France. These guidelines were developed from the 2009 WHO treatment algorithm for adult PAH patients and modified based on the experience of experts in pediatric PH.

Prostacyclin Analogues

Pediatric patients at higher risk of clinical deterioration should be considered for more aggressive treatment, including the possibility of continuous intravenous infusion therapy. Clinical signs associated with higher risk of deterioration are similar to those of adult patients and include poor functional capacity or failure to thrive, rapid progression of symptoms, clinical evidence of right heart failure or severely enlarged right ventricle or pericardial effusion on echocardiogram, syncope, or increased brain natriuretic peptide (BNP) levels. A high mPAP to systemic artery pressure ratio (>0.75) also predicts a poor prognosis as does right atrial pressure >10 mm Hg and PVRI >20 Wood units.

Epoprostenol is a potent vasodilator that is administered by continuous intravenous infusion. The prostacyclin analogue treprostinil has a longer half-life than epoprostenol and can be administered as a continuous intravenous or subcutaneous infusion. It can also be given via the inhalational route in combination with orally active PAH medications. Iloprost is another prostacyclin analog than can be given by intravenous infusion or inhalation, although only the later route is approved in the United States.[16,23]

Endothelin Receptor Antagonist

Endothelin-1 is a naturally occurring peptide synthesized by vascular endothelial cells that is a potent vasoconstrictor.[23,24] Endothelin is present at elevated concentrations in the plasma and lung tissue of patients with PAH and correlates with disease severity.[24] Two receptors, ET-A and ET-B have been identified and mediate the vascular effects of endothelin-1. Bosentan is an oral endothelin receptor antagonist (ERA) that binds to both ET-A and ET-B receptors.[23] Other endothelin receptor antagonists include ambrisentan (selective type A endothelin-1 antagonist) and macitentan (dual receptor antagonist).[23]

Phosphodiesterase Inhibitors

The vasodilatation effect of NO is mediated by cGMP. In the lung, the primary mechanism of cGMP metabolism is degradation by PDE5.[23] In patients with PAH, there is evidence that pulmonary NO synthesis is impaired and PDE5 activity is increased. [25] Sildenafil is a selective PDE5 inhibitor that can enhance pulmonary vasodilatation by slowing the degradation of cGMP.[23] It was the first PDE5 inhibitor to be approved for the treatment of PAH. Other PDE5 inhibitors that have been used for the treatment of PAH include tadalafil and vardenafil, although vardenafil is not approved for treatment of PAH in the United States.

The use of PDE5 inhibitors, specifically sildenafil in children, has been questioned due to the results of the STARTS-1 and -2 studies (Sildenafil in Treatment-Naive Children With Pulmonary Arterial Hypertension). These studies were worldwide randomized, double-blind, placebo-controlled studies in which children aged 1-17 with PAH were randomized to one of three doses of oral sildenafil (low, 10 mg; medium, 10 to 40 mg; or high, 20 to 80 mg) or placebo, 3 times

13

daily. The estimated mean ± standard error percentage change in pVO_2 for the combined treatment groups vs placebo was 7.7±4.0% (95% CI: -0.2% to 15.6%; $P=0.056$). Although a strong trend was seen favoring sildenafil, the results of the primary outcome measure were not statistically significant from placebo. In addition, there were more deaths in patients given the higher doses of sildenafil (HR 3.95; 95% CI: 1.46-10.65) for high- vs low-dose and 1.92 (95% CI: 0.65-5.65) for medium- vs low-dose.[26,27]

Review of these data led to a recommendation by the European Medicines Agency for the use of sildenafil at a dose of 10 mg 3 times daily for weight <20 kg and 20 mg 3 times daily for weight >20 kg, and a later warning against the use of higher doses. However, in August 2012, the FDA released a warning against the use of sildenafil in patients with PAH between the ages of 1 to 17 years.

Children who deteriorate on either an ERA or a PDE5 inhibitor may benefit from combination therapy with both agents or the addition of a prostacyclin analogue to their oral medical regimen.

Adjuvant Therapies

In addition to specific PAH medications, several other therapies are often used in the management of pediatric patients with PAH and should be considered on an individual basis.

Oxygen supplementation alleviates arterial hypoxemia and opposes the vasoconstriction caused by hypoxemia.[18] Children with PAH should be given oxygen as needed to maintain oxygen saturation in the mid to upper 90% range. Careful assessment for nocturnal hypoxemia should be performed including overnight oximetry or baseline sleep study if other signs of sleep disordered breathing are encountered. The use of digoxin can help improve cardiac output in patients with heart failure.[16] Diuretics may reduce symptoms of right side heart failure (eg, hepatic venous congestion).

Warfarin is recommended for adult patients with IPAH who are not at increased risk of bleeding. It may be beneficial in children with IPAH as well, particularly if they are at increased risk of thromboembolism, but it has not been as well studied.[28]

Atrial Septostomy

Atrial septostomy may be considered in patients who have severe right ventricular failure or recurrent syncope as a temporary method of unloading.[3,28]

Lung Transplantation

Lung transplantation is reserved for patients with severe PH who are not responding to any of the above mentioned treatments.

The World Symposium on Pulmonary Hypertension 2013 Consensus Pediatric IPAH/FPAH Treatment Algorithm is shown in **Figure 13.2**.

Key Points

- The etiology of pediatric PAH differs from adult PAH in that the most common causes are IPAH, HPAH, and PAH associated with congenital heart disease.
- In the newborn, PH is usually caused by PPHN or developmental lung disease such as congenital diaphragmatic hernia or bronchopulmonary dysplasia.
- Early diagnosis and treatment are important to prevent end organ damage and to improve functional capacity and survival.
- Cardiac catheterization is needed to confirm the diagnosis of PAH, determine disease etiology and severity, and assess pulmonary vasodilator response.

13

Medical treatment of pediatric PH is modeled after treatment algorithms designed for adult patients. Further studies are needed to determine the most appropriate treatment strategies for PAH in children.

FIGURE 13.2 — World Symposium on Pulmonary Hypertension 2013 Consensus Pediatric IPAH/FPAH Treatment Algorithm

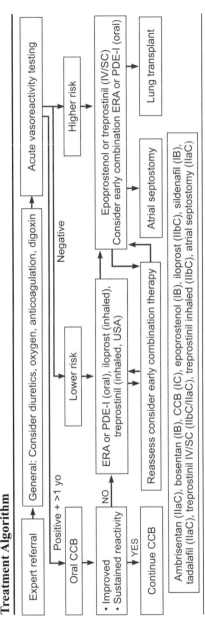

Use of all agents is considered off-label in children aside from sildenafil in Europe. Dosing recommendations per European approved dosing for children.

Ivy DD, et al. *J Am Coll Cardiol*. 2014;62(25 suppl):D117-D126.

REFERENCES

1. McLaughlin VV, McGoon MD. Pulmonary arterial hypertension. *Circulation*. 2006;114:1447-1431.

2. Walsh-Sukys MC, Tyson JE, Wright, LL, et al. Persistent pulmonary hypertension of the newborn in the era before nitric oxide: practice variation and outcomes. *Pediatrics* 2000;105;14-20.

3. Rothstein R, Paris Y, Quizon A. Pulmonary hypertension. *Pediatr Rev*. 2009;30(2);39-45.

4. Cabral JE, Belik J. Persistent pulmonary hypertension of the newborn: recent advances in pathophysiology and treatment. *J Pediatr (Rio J)*. 2013;89(3):226-242.

5. Steinhorn RH. Neonatal pulmonary hypertension. *Pediatr Crit Care Med*. 2010;11(2 suppl):S79-S84.

6. van Loon RL, Roofthooft MT, Hillege HL, et al. Pediatric pulmonary hypertension in the Netherlands: epidemiology and characterization during the period 1991 to 2005. *Circulation*. 2011;124:1744-1764.

7. Moledina S, Hislop AA, Foster H, Schulze-Neick I, Haworth SG. Childhood idiopathic pulmonary arterial hypertension: a national cohort study. *Heart*. 2010;96;1401-1406.

8. Ivy DD, Abman SH, Barst RJ, et al. Pediatric pulmonary hypertension. *J Am Coll Cardiol*. 2013;62(25 suppl):D117-D126.

9. Berger RM, M. Beghetti M, Humpl T, et al. Clinical features of paediatric pulmonary hypertension: a registry study. *Lancet*. 2012;379:537-546.

10. Widlitz A, Barst RJ. Pulmonary arterial hypertension in children. *Eur Respir J*. 2003;21(1):155-176.

11. Rich S, Rabinovitch M. Diagnosis and treatment of secondary (non-category 1) pulmonary hypertension. *Circulation*. 2008;118(21):2190-2199.

12. Deng Z, Morse JH, Slager SL, et al. Familial primary pulmonary hypertension (gene PPH1) is caused by mutations in the bone morphogenetic protein receptor-II gene. *Am J Hum Genet*. 2000;67(3):737-744.

13. Firth AL, Mandel J, Yuan JX. Idiopathic pulmonary arterial hypertension. *Dis Model Mech*. 2010;3(5-6):268-273.

14. Christman BW, McPherson CD, Newman JH, et al. An imbalance between the excretion of thromboxane and prostacyclin metabolites in pulmonary hypertension. *N Engl J Med*. 1992;327(2):70-75.

13

15. Han MK, McLaughlin VV, Criner GJ, Martinez FJ. Pulmonary diseases and the heart. *Circulation.* 2007;116(25):2992-3005.

16. McLaughlin VV, Archer SL, Badesch DB, et al; ACCF/AHA. ACCF/AHA 2009 expert consensus document on pulmonary hypertension: a report of the American College of Cardiology Foundation Task Force on Expert Consensus Documents and the American Heart Association: developed in collaboration with the American College of Chest Physicians, American Thoracic Society, Inc., and the Pulmonary Hypertension Association. *Circulation.* 2009;119(16):2250-2294.

17. Gaude GS. Pulmonary manifestations of gastroesophageal reflux disease. *Ann Thorac Med.* 2009;4(3):115-123.

18. Nauser TD, Stites SW. Diagnosis and treatment of pulmonary hypertension. *Am Fam Physician.* 2001;63(9):1789-1798.

19. Henkens IR, Scherptong RW, van Kralingen KW, Said SA, Vliegen HW. Pulmonary hypertension: the role of the electrocardiogram. *Neth Heart J.* 2008;16(7-8):250-254.

20. Jassal D, Sharma S, Maycher B. Pulmonary hypertension imaging. Medscape web site. http://emedicine.medscape.com/article/361242-overview. Published May 10, 2013. Accessed October 2, 2014.

21. Barst RJ, McGoon MD, Elliott CG, Foreman AJ, Miller DP, Ivy DD. Survival in childhood pulmonary arterial hypertension: insights from the registry to evaluate early and long-term pulmonary arterial hypertension disease management. *Circulation.* 2012;125:113-122.

22. Yung D, Widlitz AC, Rosenzweig EB, Kerstein D, Maislin G, Barst RJ. Outcomes in children with idiopathic pulmonary arterial hypertension. *Circulation.* 2004;110:660-665.

23. Duarte JD, Hanson RL, Machado RF. Pharmacologic treatments for pulmonary hypertension: exploring pharmacogenomics. *Future Cardiol.* 2013;9(3):335-349.

24. Agapitov AV, Haynes WG. Role of endothelin in cardiovascular disease. *J Renin Angiotensin Aldosterone Syst.* 2002;3(1):1-15.

25. Girgis RE, Frost AE, Hill NS, et al. Selective endothelin A receptor antagonism with sitaxsentan for pulmonary arterial hypertension associated with connective tissue disease. *Ann Rheum Dis.* 2007;66(11):1467-1472.

26. Barst RJ, Layton GR, Konourina I, Richardson H, Beghetti M, Ivy DD. STARTS-2: long-term survival with oral sildenafil monotherapy in treatment-naive patients with pediatric pulmonary arterial hypertension. *Eur Heart J.* 2012;33(suppl 1):979. Abstract.

27. Barst RJ, Ivy DD, Gaitan G, et al. A randomized, double-blind, placebo-controlled, dose-ranging study of oral sildenafil citrate in treatment-naive children with pulmonary arterial hypertension. *Circulation*. 2012;125:324.

28. Hawkins A, Tulloh R. Treatment of pediatric pulmonary hypertension. *Vasc Health Risk Manag*. 2009;5(2):509-524.

13

14 Follow-Up of the PAH Patient

by Susan Smith, ANP-BC and Alan Fein, MD

Once the diagnosis of PAH is made and a treatment plan is initiated, it is imperative that the patient be monitored closely to see how they are responding to therapy. The purpose of this chapter is to provide guidance on whether therapy is achieving clinical effectiveness and whether additional therapy should be considered. Clinical guidelines have only recently begun to address which clinical parameters should be assessed to determine if a patient is responding favorably.

In the absence of uniform agreement on a standard set of indicators, clinicians evaluating PAH patients are often left to their clinical judgment and their interpretation of an array of symptoms, signs, functional exams, hemodynamic measurements, and biomarkers to evaluate progress. This chapter will make recommendations on the approach to follow-up of patients with a diagnosis of PAH. Additionally, we will discuss psychosocial and palliative care issues that can arise and describe the role of advanced nurse practitioners and physicians assistants in managing this process.

Therapeutic goals are individually tailored based on patient needs, expectations, and life situation, and taking into account different patient populations and disease groups. Therapeutic success or clinical worsening is reflected by changes in indicators of disease severity during treatment. Although clinical trials have frequently based treatment efficacy on the improvement in 6MWD or time to clinical worsening, real world evaluations are often based on a combination of clinical indicators and the patient's perception of how

14

they are progressing. When PAH-specific medications first became available, the initial expectation was to slow disease progression. However, the development of more therapeutic options and greater experience with patient response has changed the current approach to disease management. The modern expectation for medical therapy is to restore function and pulmonary hemodynamics to as near normal as possible. In particular, modern treatment guidelines suggest that therapy be increased until improvement in WHO functional class and normalization of cardiac output at rest are achieved. The most recent treatment guidelines make a point to emphasize these more ambitious treatment goals (**Table 14.1**).

TABLE 14.1 — Proposed Goals of PAH Therapy

- Modified NYHA functional class I or II
- Normal or near normal RV size and function on echocardiogram or cardiac MRI
- Hemodynamic measurements suggesting near normal right heart function:
  - RAP <8 mm Hg
  - CI >2.5-3.0 l/min/m^2
- 6MWD 380-440 meters
- Cardiopulmonary exercise test:
  - Peak O_2 Consumption >15 mL/min/kg
  - EqCO$_2$ <45 l/min/l/min
- BNP within normal range

Adapted from McLaughlin VV, et al. *JACC*. 2013;62(25D):D73-D81.

Frequency and type of monitoring have not been clearly established by studies, but most professional guidelines recommend clinical and laboratory parameters be checked every 1 to 2 months initially or in unstable patients, then at least every 3 to 4 months going forward[1] (**Table 14.2**). The frequency and duration of follow-up after initiating a new intervention is not standardized but should be performed within 3 to 6 months.

TABLE 14.2 — Suggested Assessments and Timing for the Follow-Up of Patients With PAH

	At Baseline (prior to therapy)	Every 3-6 Months[a]	3-4 Months After Initiation or Change in Therapy	In Case of Clinical Worsening
Clinical assessment WHO-FC EKG	✓	✓	✓	✓
6MWD[b]	✓	✓	✓	✓
Cardiopulmonary exercise testing[b]	✓		✓	✓
BNP/NT-proBNP	✓	✓	✓	✓
Echocardiography	✓		✓	✓
RHC	✓[c]		✓[d]	✓

[a] Intervals should be adjusted to individual patients.
[b] Usually one of the two exercise tests is performed.
[c] Is recommended.
[d] Should be performed.

Nazzareno G, et al. *Eur Heart J.* 2009;30:2493-2537.

14

Clinical Evaluation: WHO Functional Class

Patient WHO functional class has important prognostic value. Improvement of at least one functional class (eg, from class III to II) and maintaining patients in WHO functional class I or II are strong indicators of favorable outcomes. Although determination of functional class is somewhat subjective, improving or declining functional status provides a basis for modification of pharmacologic therapy and has been used as a secondary endpoint in many clinical trials. Functional class remains a highly useful method for simple PAH assessment.

Functional Assessment PAH

The 6-minute walk distance (6MWD) test offers a low-tech and low-cost way to assess changes in functional capacity in response to medical intervention. To reduce variability between tests, the physical environment and technician training should be standardized using protocols set forth by the American Thoracic Society (ATS). Properly done, the 6MWD has been shown to provide reproducible results that provide important prognostic information. It has been the most widely used method for assessing the benefit of interventions in PAH and indeed has been the primary outcome variable for nearly every major clinical trial that has been responsible for the approval of currently available PAH-specific medications.

Two major registries have found that 6MWD predicts outcome in patients with PAH.[2,3] In one study, survival was significantly better in patients with 6MWD >380 m.[2] In another study, survival was greater in patients with 6MWD >440 m.[3] However, the test has not been validated in non-PAH pulmonary hypertension groups (Groups 2, 3, and 5) and is affected by body weight, gender, height, age, and patient motivation.[4] Goals of therapy should include improvement in 6MWD and achievement of a 6MWD greater than 380-440 feet.[5]

Cardiopulmonary Exercise Testing

Performance of cardiopulmonary exercise testing to determine maximum oxygen consumption is a standard measure in the evaluation of normal athletic performance. It has also been used to monitor patients with heart failure and PAH. The test may prove difficult to perform given the logistics of walking on a treadmill or riding a stationary bicycle, particularly in elderly patients, individuals with rheumatologic disease, or advanced right or left heart failure. This test provides helpful information regarding cardiopulmonary function in properly selected patients, but because of the limitations described above, it is infrequently employed as a measure of treatment response outside clinical research settings.

BNP/NT-proBNP

Brain natriuretic peptide (BNP) is secreted by the cardiac atria and ventricles in response to dilation of the atrium in both right and left heart failure. It is secreted as a pro-peptide (proBNP) that is metabolized to the active 32 amino acid BNP that contains the carboxy terminal and its inactive 76 amino acid N-terminal remnant NT-proBNP. Increasing plasma levels of BNP or NT-proBNP are associated with worse prognosis in PAH.[6] The NT-proBNP may provide a better indication of chronic RV overload as it is metabolized more slowly than BNP and may provide a better assessment of steady state BNP levels. Low and stable or decreasing BNP/NT-proBNP may be useful markers of successful pharmacologic intervention.[7]

In one study, survival was considerably better in patients in whom plasma BNP decreased below 180 pg/mL after 6 months of treatment.[8] Likewise, a follow-up NT-proBNP level of <1800 pg/mL was associated with better survival in PAH regardless of the value on presentation.[9] NT-proBNP is excreted by the kidney and may be elevated in patients either with concomitant renal disease or renal insufficiency alone. BNP and NT-proBNP levels also increase with age. Nonetheless, it remains a clinically useful biomarker and shows significant correlation with NYHA functional class.

Echocardiography

Echocardiography can be a very useful tool for noninvasive assessment of disease progression or cardiovascular response to specific medical therapies. Estimates of the RV systolic pressure (RVSP), which is used as a marker of pulmonary artery (PA) systolic pressure, are not precise. In a minority of patients, there is insufficient tricuspid regurgitation to measure. However, there is generally good correlation between RVSP measured by echocardiography and peak PA systolic pressures measured during right heart catheterization. Information that the echocardiogram provides about RV function is usually more important than estimates of RVSP. Measures of RV systolic function such as the tricuspid annular plan systolic excursion (TAPSE) or the Tei index.[10] and assessment of right atrial pressure (RAP) based on the collapsibility of the inferior vena cava (IVC) during inspiration are better prognostic indicators than RVSP.

Echocardiography also provides the simplest method of monitoring for the development of pericardial effusion—another indicator associated with poor prognosis.[11] Adequate echocardiography imaging may be limited in patients with obesity, chest wall disorders, or lung hyperinflation, but the echocardiogram provides useful information for most patients with PAH and is generally performed at baseline and 3 to 4 months after starting or changing therapy and then annually or bi-annually as the patient's condition stabilizes (**Table 14.2**).

Right Heart Catheterization

Three key prognostic variables, RAP, PVR, and cardiac index, permit some generalization about probable outcomes. Higher PVR and higher mean RAP predict a worse prognosis, as does a lower cardiac index. Using a formula developed from data obtained from the REVEAL registry, hemodynamic variables can be added to the other markers discussed above to provide important information regarding 1-year mortality[11] (**Figure 14.1**). Patients with high RAP or low CI are at particular danger of deterioration and should be treated most aggressively.

Right heart catheterization (RHC) provides important information regarding right- and left-sided filling pressure, cardiac output, and RV afterload that simply cannot be reliably assessed by other methods. As such, it is preferable to echocardiography or MRI for follow-up of patients with PAH. However, catheterization is invasive, expensive, and can be uncomfortable, and some patients are reluctant to repeat the procedure after initial diagnosis. Centers experienced in the care of PAH often repeat RHC every year or so in patients who appear stable or improving to confirm information provided by noninvasive testing such as 6MWD, WHO functional class, echocardiogram, and BNP.

Patients who respond well to therapy with clear signs of clinical improvement and near normalization of values obtained by noninvasive measures may not require repeat RHC. However, RHC should be considered in any patient who fails to improve or when noninvasive testing provides inconsistent or conflicting information.

14

Vaccinations

Influenza and pneumococcal vaccines should be given to prevent pulmonary infections. Early antibiotic treatment for upper respiratory infections is also war-

FIGURE 14.1 — The REVEAL Registry Risk Score Calculator and 1-Year Mortality Predictions

							SUM
WHO subgroup	CTD	+1	PoPH	+2	FPAH	+2	
Comorbidities	CKD	+1	Male, age >60	+2			
Functional Class	I	-2	III	+1	IV	+2	
Vital signs	HR >92	+1	SBP <110	+1			
6-Min walk distance	>440 m	-1	<165	+1			
BNP	<50	-2	>180	+1			
Echocardiogram	Pericardial		Effusion	+1			
PFTs	DLco >80	-1	DLco <32	+1			
Right heart catheterization	mRAP >20	+1	PVR >32 wu	+2			
						TOTAL	

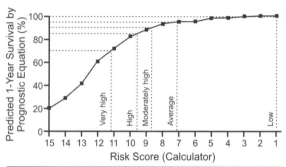

Key: BNP, plasma brain natriuretic peptide level (pg/mL); CKD, chronic kidney disease; CTD, connective tissue disease; DLco, diffusion limitation carbon monoxide (% predicted); FPAH, familial pulmonary hypertension; mRAP, mean right atrial pressure (mm Hg); PFTs, pulmonary function tests; PoPH, portopulmonary hypertension; PVR, pulmonary vascular resistance (in Woods units); SBP, systolic blood pressure (mm Hg).

Points from -2 to +2 are chosen for each row of clinical variables and placed in the last column labeled SUM. The sums of each row are added for a TOTAL point score that is used to predict 1-year mortality as shown in the graph below the table.

Modified from Benza RL, et al. *Chest*. 2012;141(2):354-362.

ranted. However, vasoconstrictive medications (ie, decongestants) should be avoided because they may increase pulmonary vascular tone.[12]

Psychosocial Issues

Anxiety and depression affect approximately one third of PH patients,[12] and the diagnosis usually confers a degree of social isolation.[13] Screening patients for depression and anxiety at regular intervals with appropriate referral to psychiatrists or psychotherapists is recommended. Activities of daily living need to be adapted to this serious chronic life-threatening disease. Encouraging patients and their family members to join patient support groups can have positive effects on coping, confidence, and outlook.[7]

Patients with PAH often benefit from participation in national organizations such as the Pulmonary Hypertension Association. The severity and rareness of this disease often leads to feelings of loneliness and despair. Realizing that thousands of patients have this disease and that many more are heavily involved in the search for better treatment and an eventual cure can help relieve much of the isolation and hopelessness experienced by many patients with PAH.

Exercise

Physical activity is encouraged for patients as long as reasonable goals are set by the patient and health care provider. Mild breathlessness is acceptable during exercise, but exertion that leads to severe breathlessness, exertional dizziness, or chest pain should be avoided.[12,13] Referral to a physical therapist or to a pulmonary rehabilitation program is advisable.[12] Studies have found that patients with severe PH on optimal stable drug therapy have significant improvement in 6MWD as well as in exercise tolerance and quality of life after participating in 15 weeks of pulmonary rehabilitation and physical therapy (see *Chapter 10*).[12,14]

14

Palliative/End of Life Care

The development of PAH-specific medications has improved the prognosis of PAH and some patients have good long-term responses, but for many patients, the clinical course of PH results in progressive deterioration. End of life is always difficult to predict; it may occur slowly due to decompensating heart failure, but sometimes occurs from sudden cardiac death. Therefore, it is important to discuss prognosis as symptoms progress and to understand each patient's preferences for advance directives.[12,15]

Opportunities to discuss prognosis should be created at the time of initial diagnosis. Recognition that cardiopulmonary resuscitation in severe PH has poor outcomes may lead patients to consider a "do not resuscitate" order and may consequently increase the chance of patients remaining in their preferred place of care at the end of life.[12,15] A palliative care referral can help ensure patients that their end of life decisions will be honored and that their symptoms of dyspnea or pain will be adequately managed. Well-informed psychological, social, and spiritual support is also vital to providing comfort at the end of life.

Air Travel

Patients with PAH should use caution when considering air travel or visits to sites at high altitude. Hypoxic pulmonary vasoconstriction can lead to acute elevations of pulmonary artery pressure and increased workload on the right ventricle. Although surveys of PH patients who participated in air travel suggest that most patients tolerate their trip without event, oxygen saturation has been shown to fall about 5% from ground levels and, in one study, symptoms of dyspnea, lightheadedness, or chest pain were reported in 11% of travelers.[16,17]

Guidelines from the American College of Cardiology Foundation and the American Heart

Association recommend supplemental oxygen for patients with PAH who have an arterial oxygen saturation of <92% on room air at sea level.[18] Guidelines from the European Society of Cardiology and European Respiratory Society recommend supplemental oxygen for PAH patients in functional class III or IV, or for those who have PaO_2 <60 mm Hg at sea level.[19] However, there is considerable variability in patient response to oxygen. Simulated high altitude testing performed in the pulmonary function lab can be used to determine an individual patient's response to hypoxia. Typically, patients are exposed to 15% oxygen to approximate an altitude of 8000 feet, the minimum cabin pressure mandated by the Federal Aviation Administration (FAA). Patients who are unable to maintain an oxygen saturation >92% or who become symptomatic should travel with supplemental oxygen. The amount of oxygen needed to maintain adequate oxygen saturation and prevent symptoms can be determined during the altitude test.

Oxygen tanks are not allowed on aircraft, but patients are permitted to use FAA-approved portable oxygen concentrators (POC). Battery life must be sufficient to provide oxygen delivery throughout the flight taking into consideration unexpected delays. Usually, multiple batteries are needed to allow for supplemental oxygen before, during, and after the flight. This requires special arrangements with the durable medical goods supplier, as many require several weeks lead time for a portable oxygen concentrator reservation to guarantee availability. Additionally, insurance coverage of portable oxygen concentrators varies, so patients need to be advised that they may have to incur out of pocket expenses if their vendor does not have a "loaner policy." Individual airlines have created airline-specific forms that must be completed and returned prior to the date of travel. Educating the patient about these issues will decrease the stress of travel.

14

Obtaining Medication

Few PAH-specific medications are available without prior authorization. Most require delivery by a specialty pharmacy and some require federally mandated lab work on a regular basis. The high cost of these medications also results in the frequent use of alternative sources of funding to make them affordable. Some manufacturers have established patient-assistance programs in the form of coupons, need-based in-company assistance, and referral to independent foundations that provide renewable grants.

Individual insurance plans each have specific guidelines that may include submission of clinical notes, laboratory data, echocardiogram, right heart catheterization, and 6MWD test results, as well as documentation of medicines tried, doses used, and patient response, along with drug-specific and plan-specific forms. Specialty pharmacies have field nurses who educate patients on device use and medication side effects. Some of these personnel are available to the patient for additional home visits or telephone consultation. For all of these reasons, centers that intend to treat more than the occasional PH patient often require the help of physician extenders such as an office nurse, nurse practitioner or physician assistant, or social worker. These personnel can be extremely helpful in making sure that new medications get started in a timely fashion and that patients are able to take advantage of any services or funding that may be available to them (see section on advanced care practitioners below).

Lung Transplantation

When maximum medical therapy fails, lung transplantation may be the only option available. In properly selected patients, lung transplantation can provide extended survival and marked improvement in functional capacity. Patients are not candidates for transplantation during the early stages of disease and usually are not presented for evaluation until all treatments have failed to show improvement. However, lung transplantation should be discussed and referrals made before the patient becomes too ill.[12,20]

In general, patients are usually considered for lung transplant evaluation when they reach functional class III or IV and have not improved on prostacyclin infusion therapy. However, full evaluation, including the assessment and resolution of socioeconomic issues can take months to accomplish and the wait time for a donor lung varies considerably depending on the patient's clinical parameters and geographic location. Therefore, it is prudent to begin the evaluation process early. Practitioners who care for PAH patients should establish a referral relationship with a lung transplant center that is experienced in transplanting patients with this disease.

Role of Advanced Care Practitioner

Many programs rely on an interdisciplinary team approach with strong collaboration between physicians of different specialties, especially rheumatologists, pulmonologists, and cardiologists. The advanced-practice nurse often plays a key role in coordination and communication between various medical team members and patients and families, and may serve as the first line of contact. Additionally, advanced-practice nurses and physician assistants frequently provide education to patients and caregivers regarding pathophysiology, progression, and treatment of PAH, as well as medication side effects.

Interdisciplinary team collaboration is needed to monitor medication efficacy, disease progression, and manage care. Nurse practitioners have both diagnostic and clinical management roles. They often obtain a complete history and physical exam, order laboratory and diagnostic testing, and make appropriate referrals to other members of the multidisciplinary team. Patient and family/caregiver education is an important role of

14

the nurse practitioner or physician assistant (**Table 14.3** and **Table 14.4**).[12]

TABLE 14.3 — Educational Role of the Advance Care Practitioner

- Disease pathology, signs of deterioration, and progression
- Medication use, dosing, compliance, device management, titration schedules
- Nutritional counseling
- Weight management
- Lifestyle changes
- Exercise programs
- Patient coping techniques/stress management
- Caregiver support
- Referral to local support group
- Information on financial assistance programs
- Discuss reasoning and need for follow-up testing
- Safe management of oxygen at home
- Smoking cessation
- Avoid decongestant use

TABLE 14.4 — Clinical Management Role of the Advance Care Patient

- History and physical
- Order initial and follow-up laboratory and diagnostic testing
- Order medication
- Obtain prior authorizations for medications
- Coordinate collaboration within multidisciplinary team
- Order durable medical equipment (DME)
- Follow-up after medication initiation or change

- Due to the progressive nature of PAH, close follow-up with regularly scheduled testing is warranted.
- Serial assessments using multiple modalities are essential with the goal of returning right heart function, pulmonary hemodynamics, and functional capacity to as near normal as possible.
- In addition to response to medical therapy, patients psychosocial and end of life needs should be addressed.
- An interdisciplinary team, consisting of multiple medical specialties and advanced care practitioners, helps to ensure successful patient management and adequate support to patients and families.

14

REFERENCES

1. Nazzareno G, Hoeper MM, Humbert M, et al. Guidelines for the diagnosis and treatment of pulmonary hypertension. *Eur Heart J*. 2009;30:2493-2537.

2. Benza RL, Miller DP, Comberg-Maitland M, et al Predicting survival in pulmonary arterial hypertension: insight from the Registry to Evaluate Early and Lung-Term pulmonary arterial hypertension Disease management (REVEAL). *Circulation*. 2010:122:164-172.

3. Sitbon O, Humbert M, Nunes H, et al. Long-term intravenous epoprostenol infusion in primary pulmonary hypertension: prognostic factors ad survival. *J Am Coll Cardiol*. 2002;40:780-788.

4. ATS Committee on Proficiency Standards for Clinical Pulmonary Function Laboratories. ATS statement: guidelines for the six-minute walk test. *Am J Respir Crit Care Med*. 2002;166:111-117.

5. McLaughlin VV, Gaine SP, Howard LS, et al. Treatment goals of pulmonary hypertension. *JACC*. 2013;62 suppl 25:D73-D81.

6. Williams MH, Handler CE, Akram R, et al. Role of N-terminal brain natriuretic peptide (N-TproBNP) in scleroderma-associated pulmonary arterial hypertension. *Eur Heart J*. 2006;27:1485-1494.

7. Galie N, Hoeper MM, Humbert M, et al; ESC Committee for Practice Guidelines (CPG). Guidelines for diagnosis and treatment of pulmonary hypertension: the Task Force for the Diagnosis and Treatment of Pulmonary Hypertension of the European Society of Cardiology (ESC) and the European Respiratory Society (ERS), endorsed by the International Society of Heart and Lung Transplantation (ISHLT). *Eur Heart J*. 2009;30(20):2493-2537.

8. Nagaya N, Nishikimi T, Uematsu M, et al. Plasma brain natriuretic peptide as a prognostic indicator in patients with primary pulmonary hypertension. *Circulation*. 2000;102(8):865-870.

9. Nickel N, Golpon H, Greer M, et al. The prognostic impact of follow up assessments in patients with idiopathic pulmonary arterial hypertension. *Eur Respir J*. 2012;39:589-596.

10. Yeo TC, Dujardin KS, Tei C, Mahoney DW, McGoon MD, Seward JB. Value of a Doppler-derived index combining systolic and diastolic time intervals in predicting outcome in primary pulmonary hypertension. *Am J Cardiol*. 1998;81(9):1157-1161.

11. Benza RL, Gomberg-Maitland M, Miller DP, et al. The REVEAL Registry risk score calculator in patients newly diagnosed with pulmonary arterial hypertension. *Chest.* 2012;141(2):354-362.

12. Tartavoulle TM. Evaluation and management of the adult patient with pulmonary hypertension. *JNP.* 2011;7(5):409-416.

13. Loewe B, Graefe K, Ufer C, et al. Anxiety and depression in patients with pulmonary hypertension. *Psychosom Med.* 2004;66(6):831-836.

14. Mereles D, Ehlken N, Kreuscher S, et al. Exercise and respiratory training improve exercise capacity and quality of life in patients with severe chronic pulmonary hypertension. *Circulation.* 2006;114(14):1482-1489.

15. Gin-Sing W. Pulmonary arterial hypertension: a multidisciplinary approach to care. *Nurs Stand.* 2010;24(38):40-47.

16. Roubinian N, Elliott CG, Barnett CF, et al. Effects of commercial air travel on patients with pulmonary hypertension air travel and pulmonary hypertension. *Chest.* 2012;142(4):885-892.

17. Thamm M, Voswinckel R, Tiede H, et al. Air travel can be safe and well tolerated in patients with clinically stable pulmonary hypertension. *Pulm Circ.* 2011;1(2):239-243.

18. Galiè N, Hoeper MM, Humbert M, et al. Guidelines for the diagnosis and treatment of pulmonary hypertension: the Task Force for the Diagnosis and Treatment of Pulmonary Hypertension of the European Society of Cardiology (ESC) and the European Respiratory Society (ERS), endorsed by the International Society of Heart and Lung Transplantation (ISHLT). *Eur Heart J.* 2009;30(20):2493-2537.

19. McLaughlin VV, Archer SL, Badesch DB, et al American College of Cardiology Foundation Task Force on Expert Consensus Documents; American Heart Association; American College of Chest Physicians; American Thoracic Society, Inc; Pulmonary Hypertension Association. ACCF/AHA 2009 expert consensus document on pulmonary hypertension a report of the American College of Cardiology Foundation Task Force on Expert Consensus Documents and the American Heart Association developed in collaboration with the American College of Chest Physicians; American Thoracic Society, Inc.; and the Pulmonary Hypertension Association. *J Am Coll Cardiol.* 2009;53(17):1573-1619.

20. Hayes GB. *Pulmonary Hypertension: A Patient's Survival Guide.* Silver Spring, MD: Pulmonary Hypertension Association; 2010.

14

15 Abbreviations/Acronyms

6MWD	6-minute walk distance
ACC	American College of Cardiology
AHA	American Heart Association
AIDS	acquired immune deficiency syndrome
ALK1	activin receptor-like kinase type 1
ANP	atrial natriuretic peptide
APAH	associated pulmonary arterial hypertension
APAH-CHD	pulmonary arterial hypertension associated with congenital heart disease
ARDS	acute respiratory distress syndrome
ASD	atrial septal defect
ATS	American Thoracic Society
AVR	aortic valve replacement
AVT	acute vasodilator testing
BAS	balloon atrial septostomy
BGA	blood gas analysis
BMI	body mass index
BMPR2	bone morphogenic receptor type 2 receptor
BNP	brain natriuretic peptide
BPM	beats per minute
BREATHE	Bosentan Randomized Trial of Endothelin Antagonist Therapy [trial]
Ca	calcium
$[Ca^{2+}]_i$	intracellular calcium
CCB	calcium channel blocker
CCHS	congenital central hypoventilation syndrome
CDC	Centers for Disease Control and Prevention

cGMP	cyclic guanosine monophosphate
CHD	congenital heart disease
CHEST	Chronic Thromboembolic Pulmonary Hypertension sGC-Stimulator Trial
CI	confidence interval
CMR	cardiac magnetic resonance
CNP	C-type natriuretic peptide
COPD	chronic obstructive pulmonary disease
CPAP	continuous positive airway pressure
CT	computed tomography
CTD	connective tissue disease
CTEPH	chronic thromboembolic pulmonary hypertension
CVP	central venous pressure
CXR	chest x-ray
D$_{LCO}$	carbon monoxide diffusing capacity
DME	durable medical equipment
DPAH	drug-induced pulmonary arterial hypertension
EARLY	Endothelin Antagonist Trial in Mildly Symptomatic Pulmonary Arterial Hypertension Patients [trial]
ECMO	extracorporeal membrane oxygenation
EF	ejection fraction
EKG	electrocardiogram
eNOS	endothelial nitric oxide synthase
ERA	endothelin receptor antagonist
ESC/ERS	European Society of Cardiology and European Respiratory Society
ET	endothelin
ET-1	endothelin-1
ET-A	endothelin A [receptor]
ET-B	endothelin B [receptor]
FDA	Food and Drug Administration

FEV$_1$	forced expiratory volume in 1 second
FPAH	familial pulmonary arterial hypertension
FVC	forced vital capacity
GDE	goal-directed echocardiography
GERD	gastroesophageal reflux disease
GMP	guanosine monophosphate
HAART	highly active antiretroviral therapy
HIV	human immunodeficiency virus
HPAH	heritable pulmonary arterial hypertension
HR	heart rate
HRCT	high-resolution computed tomography
ICU	intensive care unit
iNO	inhaled nitric oxide
IPAH	idiopathic pulmonary arterial hypertension
IPH	idiopathic pulmonary hypertension
IV/i.v.	intravenous
IVC	inferior vena cava
LFT	liver function test
LPV	lung protective ventilation
LV	left ventricle
LVEDP	left ventricular end-diastolic pressure
m	meter
MAO	monoamine oxidase
MAP	mean systemic arterial pressure
MID	minimal important difference
min	minute(s)
MLC	myosin light chain
MLCPase	myosin light chain phosphotase
mPAP	mean pulmonary arterial pressure
MRI	magnetic resonance imaging
MVR	mitral valve replacement

15

NAION	nonarteritic ischemic optic neuropathy
NICE	National Institute for Health and Care Excellence
NO	nitric oxide
NOTT	Nocturnal Oxygen Therapy in Hypoxemic Chronic Obstructive Lung Disease Trial
NPR-A	natriuretic peptide receptor-A
NSAID	nonsteroidal anti-inflammatory drug
NSIP	nonspecific idiopathic pneumonia
NT-proBNP	N-terminal of the prohormone brain natriuretic peptide
NYHA	New York Heart Association
OR	odds ratio
PA	pulmonary artery
PAC	pulmonary artery catheter
PAH	pulmonary arterial hypertension
PAP	pulmonary artery pressure
PATENT	Pulmonary Arterial Hypertension sGC-Stimulator Trial
PAVM	pulmonary arteriovenous malformation
PAWP	pulmonary artery wedge pressure
PCA	prostacyclin analogue
PCH	pulmonary capillary hemangiomatosis
PCWP	pulmonary capillary wedge pressure
PDA	patent ductus arteriosus
PDE	phosphodiesterase
PDE2	phosphodiesterase type-2
PDE5	phosphodiesterase type-5
PDE5I	phosphodiesterase type-5 inhibitor
PE	pulmonary embolism
PEA	pulmonary endarterectomy
PEA	pulseless electrical activity
PEEP	positive end-expiratory pressure
PFT	pulmonary function test

pGC	particulate guanylate cyclase
PGI_2	prostacyclin
PH	pulmonary hypertension
PHIRST	Pulmonary Arterial Hypertension and Response to Tadalafil [trial]
PKG	protein kinase G
PoPH	portopulmonary hypertension
PPHN	persistent pulmonary hypertension of the newborn
PPV	pulse pressure variation
PVOD	pulmonary veno-occlusive disease
PVR	pulmonary vascular resistance
PVRI	pulmonary vascular resistance index
RA	right atrium
RAP	right atrial pressure
RCT	randomized controlled trial
REMS	Risk Evaluation and Mitigation Strategies
REVEAL	Registry to Evaluate Early and Long-Term PAH Management
RHC	right heart catheterization
RTI	reverse transcriptase inhibitor
RV	right ventricle
RVAD	right ventricular assist device
RVEDP	right ventricular end-diastolic pressure
RVOT	right ventricular outflow tract
RVSP	right ventricle systolic pressure
SBP	systolic blood pressure
s.c.	subcutaneous
SERAPHIN	Study with an Endothelin Receptor Antagonist in Pulmonary Arterial Hypertension to Improve Clinical Outcome
sGC	soluble guanylate cyclase
sGCS	soluble guanylate cyclase stimulator
SLE	systemic lupus erythematosus

15

sPAP	pulmonary artery systolic pressure
SSRI	selective serotonin reuptake inhibitor
SUPER	Sildenafil Use in Pulmonary Arterial Hypertension [trial]
SV	stroke volume
SvO_2	mixed venous oxygen saturation
TAPSE	tricuspid annular plane systolic excursion
TGF-β	transforming growth factor
TR	tricuspid regurgitation
TRV	tricuspid regurgitation velocity
TXA_2	thromboxane
ULN	upper limit of normal
V/Q	ventilation/perfusion
V-A ECMO	venoarterial extracorporeal membrane oxygenation
VE/VCO_2	ventilator equivalents for carbon dioxide
VMI	ventricular mass index
VO_2	oxygen consumption
VSD	ventricular septal defect
WHO	World Health Organization
WHO-FC	World Health Organization functional class
wk	week(s)
x-ray	chest radiograph
yo	year(s) old

Note: PH stands for pulmonary hypertension;
PAH for pulmonary arterial hypertension.
Page numbers in *italics* indicate figures.
Page numbers followed by a "t" indicate tables.
Clinical trials are indexed under the acronym of the name.

16

16

16

16

16

16

16

16

16

325

16

16

16

16

16